Intertwined

Gavin S. Johnson
Intertwined

ISBN 979-8-89950-157-9

Spines

INTERTWINED

A JOURNEY INTO THE HEART OF ONE OF THE WORLD'S MOST INTERESTING CITIES FROM A UNIQUE PERSPECTIVE...

GAVIN S. JOHNSON

Contents

Preface

A lot has happened in the last 2 decades…The Indian Ocean tsunami, Hurricane Katrina and its aftermath, BP oil spill, numerous earthquakes in diverse places, the Japan nuclear disaster, the Covid 19 pandemic, and of all things a terror attack in my hometown… And we have been foretold that these are the beginning of sorrows… The world is on fire these days as we can see globally. Being the son of an older jazz musician and a younger mother, growing up in New Orleans, I've seen the world from a unique perspective early on in my life. I see the current state of everything and feel I'm prepared to see what's to come no matter how bad it gets. My experience of being stranded with my elderly father at work in a prison for Hurricane Katrina was quite traumatic, but we made it out alive somehow. Being surrounded by water, rioting prisoners, desperate civilians, and dramatic uncertainty… It opened my eyes to how bad things can get when in a dire situation. We certainly didn't plan for what unfolded but in a way I'm ok with what happened. I know I can survive and function in an apocalyptic type of event which I feel will come in my lifetime. I have had this dream and vision many times…

Fast forward 20 years later and I've now gone into the underbelly of New Orleans to see some very unique things. Being a healthcare provider offers up some interesting situations that the everyday person wouldn't see. I've literally been in a crack house, a mansion, a prison cell and a rehab room in the same day. Crazy… I know, but it's quite interesting. I was amazed how they can all be *intertwined* at times. I don't want to spoil the story for you too much, but I did see a rehab patient that was also an inmate that had a family member that I saw that same day on a home health visit.

This a journey that will take a step back in time as well, 20 years ago to an unbelievable situation to a unique view of how certain segments of our world live in a city that was tailor made for this social experiment.

The end of 2024 and beginning of 2025 saw a slew of worldwide events take place in the city from a Taylor Swift multi concert, to the Sugar Bowl, to a disastrous New Year's Day Terror Attack on Bourbon Street, and another record tying successful Super Bowl. The countless festivals, restaurants, parties, Mardi Gras and so on that was filled with different scenarios. I only set out on this journey to document the drug and crime crisis this country was in and ended up in situations I never imagined…

Part One

INTERTWINED...

A DIFFERENT LOOK INTO ANOTHER SIDE OF ONE OF THE WORLD'S MOST INTERESTING CITIES...

Wow... Where on earth has the time slipped away? Here we are in 2023, and the drug and crime crises in urban America are spiraling to unimaginable lows. Cities like New Orleans are grappling with a grisly surge of violent offenses and an overwhelming wave of drug-related mayhem. My intrigue has been bubbling up over the past couple of years, fueled by the escalating crime situation in our nation. Opioids, Benzodiazepines, fentanyl, brazen carjackings, domestic abuse, the border turmoil with illegal crossings... I felt compelled to witness it all myself. Just how dire can the reality be? So, I'm heading back to work part-time as a nurse at the Orleans Justice Center—that's right, the place that used to be known as the Orleans Parish Criminal Sheriff's Office, now under new management, and it feels like I'm stepping into a whole new universe. The shifts since I first joined the ranks in 2003, weathered through Hurricane Katrina, left as a part-time nurse in 2009, and now returning in 2023, are nothing short of astounding! Back then, I was navigating a divorce and needed a clean slate in my life! Now, I'm re-entering the arena as a quasi-undercover investigator, seeking to uncover the truths lurking beneath the surface of this chaotic landscape.

I have to admit, when I first set off on this quest, I never expected to find myself chronicling a terrorist attack on New Year's Day 2025 in the heart of New Orleans. It was a time when I believed I was merely finalizing the pages of this book, only to have the unthinkable crash into reality. That ominous night, I lingered in downtown, soaking in the atmosphere until nearly 10:30 p.m. The notion that chaos was already brewing, ready to unleash at any moment during that vibrant evening, is a difficult burden to process. Below, you'll find a couple of links that provide further insights into the harrowing events, including a family interview and strategies for ensuring safety ahead of the 2025 Super Bowl and the future. Here are the details: (https://www.wdsu.com/artice/neworleans-terror-attack-jabbar-live-updates/63320965, https/x.-com/nolanews/status/1876132916603826220?s=12, https://www.nola.com/news/isis-new-orleans-bourbon-street-terrorist/article_fcbc1c80-ced0-11ef-8499-07980e0b5795.html)

As of January 21st, 2025, city officials made an urgent appeal to the Department of Homeland Security and successfully attained SEAR 1 safety measures status. "Per the Homeland Security website, SEAR 1 encompasses significant events that hold national and/or international significance, warranting extensive federal interagency backing. This designation would allocate federal funding for safety enhancements and facilitate the involvement of experts to pinpoint vulnerabilities within the city's security framework. The SEAR 1 designation also entails the deployment of bomb-sniffing dog units, comprehensive cybersecurity assessments, security screenings at key sites, aerial surveillance, and tactical response teams…" Military vehicles were strategically stationed around the Superdome, a striking sight indeed. On a lighter note, New Orleans and the entire region found themselves enveloped in an unexpected phenomenon—SNOW! And it was a considerable amount! Ah, this is how we roll down here, lol.

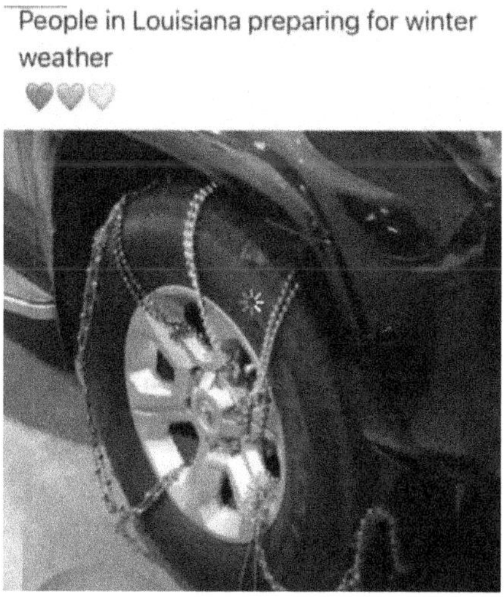

A lot is going on in the city these days! Anyway, enough of that; back to the matter at hand...

As you will discover, today's urban criminals are not only younger but also audacious, pushing boundaries like never before. The drug issue has spiraled out of control, far worse than I had anticipated. I felt an undeniable urge to return, driven by a personal story that needs sharing, and, serendipitously, the timing couldn't be more perfect. Upon my arrival, I reached out to a couple of old friends who manage a home health agency. Having assisted them with marketing from 2015 to 2017, I was curious to see if they required any nurses. My intention was to refresh my nursing skills, which had grown rusty after years away from tasks like venipuncture, wound care, and administering injections. Fortuitously, they were indeed in need, a reflection of the nationwide nursing shortage that has become a pressing issue. Little did I know that this endeavor would lead me to a couple of patients in my rotation who, by a curious twist of fate (or perhaps by design, as I'm convinced much in life is not merely coincidence—lol), once belonged to the New Orleans Criminal Sheriff's Office in years past. More on that later.

A few months into my social experiment, I found myself picking up a PRN (part-time) job at a relatively prominent rehabilitation facility in the vibrant heart of New Orleans. I aimed to gain a first-hand glimpse into the substance abuse challenges that grip our society, with a specific focus on the complex ways they manifest here. The visibility of the cycle—from incarceration to rehab as a means to dodge a prison sentence, blending the lives of civilians and those grappling with addiction—compelled me to explore the blurred lines between sobriety and relapse. It struck me that for those confined within jail walls, remorse for their choices might not signify they've truly reached rock bottom; often, it becomes a mere stop on their challenging journey. New Orleans stands as a unique city, where one might visit a patient living in a mansion in Uptown, only to turn the corner and encounter another whose dwelling resembles a borderline "crack house." It's hard to believe, yet I'd assert that this phenomenon is unlike anywhere else in the country. For those familiar with this city's fabric, it resonates deeply; for those yet to experience it, a visit will surely show these contrasts. This wasn't part of my original plan, but as I navigated the orientation at the prison, the parallels between seeking help for addiction, serving time for drug-related offenses, and the intersection with the city's residents in need of home health care became evident. What struck me most were the shocking, grim realities faced by those living in dire poverty, highlighting an unforgiving chasm between the fortunate and the less fortunate.

An intriguing observation struck me during my time at the rehabilitation facility… I began to notice a curious pattern: a striking number of patients were left-handed when it came time to sign their medication charts. Why this caught my attention, I couldn't quite pinpoint, but it nagged at me. It often happened as I would hand them the pen, my instinct leading me to offer it toward their right hand, only to watch as they confidently grabbed it with their left. The way many of these left-handed individuals wrote—with their hands subtly angled—was undeniably distinctive. Intrigued, I delved into some research and found that only about 10% of the global population is left-handed. Yet, at my facility, nearly 40% of the patients were part of this minority. I couldn't shake the feeling that this wasn't mere coincidence. Digging deeper, I stumbled upon the startling revelation that left-handed individuals face a greater likelihood of grappling with substance abuse issues and may be more susceptible to mental health disorders. Fascinating… Who would have guessed? It seems intertwined, with the developmental intricacies of left-handed brains playing a role, compounded by socio-economic factors that increase the prevalence of addiction concerns. Additionally, I found that many elite athletes—boxers, tennis players, major league baseball players, and others—tend to skew left-handed as well.

Part of my research has uncovered a fascinating trend: as previously noted, left-handed individuals make up about 10% of the global population, yet they account for a striking 30% of Major League Baseball players, 20% of professional boxers, and a considerable number of top-tier athletes in both professional tennis tours. The statistics are intriguing, and they suggest something deeper at play. Therefore, if there are any left-handed individuals in your circle grappling with substance abuse challenges, or if you notice younger teens on the brink of such paths, it's wise to keep a vigilant eye on them. It's important to remind them to stay alert, as the data suggests they might be more vulnerable to addiction. I realize this might sound implausible, but the prevalence of left-handed people receiving treatment at my current facility is hard to overlook. Now, let's return to the present moment.

Chapter 1

NOW vs THEN

It feels like only yesterday when I was nervously perched at the edge of my seat in my final semester of nursing school, waiting for some elusive job recruiter to sweep in and enlighten us about our futures. Whispers circulated about the unknown figure, but nothing could have prepared me for the moment when a doctor, accompanied by two poised nurses, entered our classroom. "Greetings, everyone… I'm Doctor… and I serve as the Medical Director at the Orleans Parish Criminal Sheriff's Office.These are my colleagues, and we're here to present a unique opportunity for you to work within the prison system." My heart raced—this was certainly not what I'd envisioned for myself. The thought of nursing in a prison had never entered my mind; I had my sights set on a corporate career in pharmaceutical sales, hoping to eventually care for my aging father, who was 81 at that time. He had me at the seasoned age of 50, while my mother was just 23… But that's a story for another time!

Every now and then, he would lean in, being the character that he was, and say, "Son, just promise me this: never put me in a nursing home…" His unique spirit lingers in my mind like a favorite song, and there's a quiet ache in my heart for the stories we shared. Yet, I cling to the hope of reuniting with him someday. As I settled into my seat, absorbing the presentation unfolding before me, I felt a surprising curiosity wash over me about the opportunity being laid out. With a college degree in hand and a few years of sales experience tucked under my belt, here I was in the final weeks of nursing school, intrigued by a doctor's words about the unconventional life of working behind bars. Reflecting on my journey, I realized that my life had always danced to a different beat, and suddenly, this prospect didn't seem so peculiar after all.

Back to the doctor. He presented a persuasive argument for working at the prison, outlining the advantages with the flair of a salesman. As I sat there, contemplating my upcoming wedding in June of 2003, a chill ran through the winter of 2002 as I absorbed the enticing perks of the job— an impressive 12-year pension plan, remarkable health benefits, a 401k, ample PTO, and sick leave. It painted a picture of opportunity that was hard to ignore. But first, the hurdle of nursing school awaited me, followed by the daunting state board exam, a necessary gauntlet to entering the nursing field. But I triumphed; I passed the exam in March of 2003, and with my wedding in June on the horizon, I set forth on my new journey in correctional nursing.

My inaugural task in orientation plunged me into the world of "sick call" on the 10th floor of the House of Detention ("HOD") building. This particular floor housed both male and female psychiatric patients, a realm where shadows mingled with the flicker of hope. Beneath the 10th, the 7th floor contained step-down psychiatric inmates; they lacked acute crises but still clung to their psych meds, an anchor in their daily struggles. As I walked the 1st floor "Sallie Port," the air tinged with the musty scent of aged materials, and memories of past lives echoed in the environmental supply area. Constructed in 1967, this building bore witness to the passage of time, each brick a story; closures may come, but history lingers. Despite its closing in 2012, it still looms, its ghostly presence a stark contrast to the newer structures nearby. I'd urge you to check out this mesmerizing video that reveals the haunting depths of the HOD building, blending the eerie past with the current state of decay.

https://youtu.be/MIvOcTFKlEc?si=LLR2_tmEA0_3xcEo

The HOD is next to the municipal court building, and from what I gather, it's a historical landmark; it is likely to remain for many years ahead, impenetrable to any plans for demolition.

Back to where I was going with this… as I walked into this dilapidated old building, I remember asking myself, "What the hell was I doing?" Anyway, I took the elevator up to the 10th floor, got off, and walked right into the medical clinic. I introduced myself to the psychiatrist and the other two nurses there and sat down as the first inmate was brought in. She was a female, mid-30s, I believe, with a slight limp. She was an attractive blonde who ended up arguing/fighting with her boyfriend on a flight from Miami to Las Vegas, and by federal law, they were forced to land at the nearest airport, which was in New Orleans. Both were subsequently arrested and booked into Orleans Parish Prison. As she sat down in the medical clinic, she proceeded to demand her Xanax medication from the psychiatrist, among other things. He quickly shot that down and after a few more minutes, she was brought back to her cell, noticeably limping out in handcuffs. I didn't think much of it at the time and thought "this is gonna be some wild shit up here!"

After a few rounds of "sick call" evaluations, suddenly, a blood-curdling scream pierced the air, "HELP!!! HELP ME!!!!, HELP!!!!..." We exchanged anxious glances as the urgency of the charge nurse prompted her to seize the Emergency Bag, leading us swiftly to the tier where the chaos erupted. We had to stand by, waiting for the deputy to unlock the cell door, the cries echoing off the walls. To my astonishment, there was the notorious "airplane" lady sprawled on the floor, her FAKE LEG in hand, exclaiming, "I fell, and I can't get my leg to reattach!" We all struggled to suppress laughter, picturing her on that cold floor, clutching her prosthetic leg as she theatrically lamented her misfortune. It all made sense now—the limp! A wild start to my first couple of hours, wouldn't you say?

Fast forward about a year and a half, and there I was, out on the links with some friends on a balmy Friday afternoon—August 26, 2005. After finishing our round, we settled in to share a few beers and shoot the breeze. Just then, the news bulletin crackled on the screen, leading with a grim report: "Category 1 Hurricane Katrina is battering the Florida coast and is expected to move into the Gulf of Mexico, where it's likely to strengthen…" A knot tightened in my stomach; I recognized that foreboding sign—a storm seemed inevitable, and we'd been lucky to escape nature's wrath in recent years. Once we wrapped up our conversation, I picked up the phone and dialed my dad. He was 83 by then, firm in his ways and stubborn as ever. "I'm not going anywhere… How did you play today?" he asked, laughter trailing in his voice. I chuckled softly, replying, "Not too shabby, but I'm a little uneasy about this storm… You know, there's a place at the jail where civilians can stay if things get rough… It's decent enough." He dismissed the idea, and I promised to check in with him again tomorrow. I headed home to unwind with my wife, knowing I had a busy weekend ahead.

As dawn broke on Saturday morning, I was still recovering from the remnants of a sleepless night. I flicked on the television, only to be greeted by dire news: the hurricane had escalated, bearing down on New Orleans with alarming speed! My wife and I exchanged anxious glances, and it was quickly understood—she would evacuate with the dogs, no matter what. I insisted she reach out to her parents while I dialed my dad, desperately trying to persuade him to make the same choice. As a city employee and a nurse, duty bound me to report to work; the stakes were high with my nursing license on the line. There was no way I could jeopardize that. I managed to rally my wife and her family to evacuate, but convincing my dad proved to be a greater challenge. His stubbornness was palpable as he insisted he'd be fine. Eventually, I negotiated a compromise—to have him stay with me at the prison. Not the safest haven, I knew, but at least I could watch over him. People often asked how he ended up there, and now you know the story. Though I wished he'd chosen to evacuate, he reluctantly complied. We both had our opportunities to flee, and now we would face the impending storm together, paying the price for our resistance.

Now, in the year 2023, I've made a decisive move to return and take on part-time work, embarking on a journey of observation and insight in a place I left behind fourteen years ago. As I step into this role and arrive for my first day of orientation, it feels monumental; for the first time, I'm experiencing the new prison up close. Towering four stories high, the main structure stands like a fortress, its stark, looming presence contrasting with the sleek administrative side, defined by elevators that glide effortlessly to the prison's entrance. Unlike the sprawling designs of the past, where facilities sprawled aimlessly across numerous buildings and city blocks, this newer layout is refreshingly compact and remarkably efficient. In the aftermath of the Katrina days, when this system could hold around six to seven thousand inmates at its peak, the population is now a mere one thousand to twelve hundred. Whispers float through the corridors about plans to erect yet another facility across from the old HOD building—a site thick with memories, where my father and I found ourselves marooned nearly two decades ago.

In the wake of Hurricane Katrina, the pandemonium unleashed by that fateful disaster revealed a torrent of human anguish and despair, horrific beyond imagination—an event that must never be repeated! It was a complex interplay of tragic decisions and cruel chance. At first, it appeared the city had narrowly escaped the worst, but when the levees crumbled, an overwhelming deluge transformed the familiar terrain into a haunting wasteland. I can vividly recall emerging onto the second-floor mezzanine once the skies cleared, where not a single cloud dared to hang above, and the streets were mere shadows of their former selves, with hints of water. Yet, as the hours trudged forward, apocalyptic downpours engulfed the area, warping New Orleans into a surreal level of ruin, irrevocably altering the fabric of life as we once knew it.

Back to the new facility… Everything inside feels like a whole new universe. The sleek elevators hum as they whisk you upward, and the electronic glass doors slide open silently to reveal the administration floor. Badges reign supreme, granting access to every corner of this modern facility. Quite a contrast to the old clunky key locks, the dreary, worn corridors, and the musty cells of the past—it's almost comical! I remember binge-watching the Black Bird series with Taron Egerton on Netflix about a year ago, and in a gripping episode, I realized they shot much of it in the abandoned OPP (Orleans Parish Prison) complex, which has been dormant since the devastation of Hurricane Katrina! It was surreal to recognize the very hallways and spaces I had navigated countless times, bringing back a flood of memories tied to those shadowy, oppressive walls.

Anyway, I arrived on my first day of orientation and stepped into the conference room. We all introduced ourselves, and almost immediately, we were handed a drug screening device. I'd never encountered anything like it, so I looked it up later. It was called the 5 Panel InstaCube Saliva Drug Test, and to use it, you had to suck on this awkward gadget while swirling it around in your mouth to generate as much saliva as humanly possible. They even provided napkins because, let's be real, drool was pretty much guaranteed during this process, and it took a staggering 30 to 45 minutes to produce enough spit to finish the test! The results?

Instantaneous. So much for the old-school urine test, right? Just picture it: eight people sitting around a table, all of us awkwardly sucking on these tests, drooling like a bunch of kids after a popsicle! Truly, just like in 2003, this was quite the entertaining beginning to round two at this place! Next up was the Covid test. Standard fare, really… I guess this nonsense is here to stay…

Fortunately, no one faced immediate dismissal due to a failed drug test, which was a relief, so we transitioned into the orientation for WellPath Company. This is the healthcare management firm responsible for overseeing medical operations within the jail. To my surprise, they are actually a global enterprise! While their roots lie in the United States, they also manage correctional facilities in Australia! Who would have thought? It's a stark contrast to my previous experiences here. Back in 2003, the doctors, nurses, and all medical personnel were directly employed by the city and the Sheriff's Department. Now, they distinctly operate as WellPath employees, separate from the prison staff. On a side note, as I've heard from various sources, the once generous benefits associated with the job back in 2003 have vanished. Gone are the pensions, and the healthcare coverage resembles what is now the norm—less than ideal. I was taking on a PRN (part-time) role, so benefits wouldn't apply to me anyway. I must admit, the hourly wage is quite decent, which perhaps reflects the necessity of attracting healthcare workers in today's climate.

The initial hours and days unfolded smoothly. We transitioned to the training center for the new recruits aspiring to become deputies, and I began to perceive some stark contrasts from years past. As we navigated the corridor leading to the medical training section, I spotted around thirty eager recruits, each appearing no older than twenty! My astonishment was palpable. I remarked to a fellow orientee, a former deputy now pursuing nursing, about this shift. She replied, "That's the pressing issue here now… They're struggling to attract anyone but fresh-faced high school graduates."

Quite intriguing… Anyway, today marked the start of our immersion into the Wellpath systems and the protocols in medical practice. To declare it an enlightening experience would be an understatement! The complexity and breadth exceed what I had anticipated. There were a handful of systems back in 2003 through 2009, but fast forward to 2023 and it's an entirely different universe! We encountered a multitude of systems, each with unique usernames and passwords. The WellPath EMR (Electronic Medical Records) system is immense. It's a far leap from the rudimentary AS400 and paper-based charting we relied on 14 years ago. After diligently working through the 44-page "Team Member Handbook," we decided to call it a day. Little did we know, the following day would hold even greater surprises.

In 2003, Congress came together to pass the Prison Rape Elimination Act (PREA). This significant piece of legislation aimed to "provide analysis of the incidence and effects of prison rape in federal, state, and local correctional institutions, while also offering resources, information, recommendations, and funding designed to protect individuals from the horrors of prison rape." (Prison Rape Elimination Act, 2003.) To take a brief detour, it's worth noting that in 2010, the Bureau of Justice Assistance established the National PREA Resource Center. This center was dedicated to ensuring ongoing training and support for states and localities, serving as a vital hub for research and tools aimed at helping those in the field comply with federal mandates. My intention in discussing this is to illuminate the aspects of the prison system that are subject to scrutiny and regulation. For reasons that escape me, this was not on my radar two decades ago, yet it's evident that by 2023, there has been a renewed focus on these crucial issues.

As we delved into the intricacies of the PREA Act, we found ourselves in a surprising and somewhat surreal session where images of "Trans" individuals from past arrests flashed before us. The expectation was clear: as a collective, we were tasked with deciphering the biological sex of each person while also trying to understand how they identified. That hour turned into an unprecedented revelation for me! The stack of arrest records featured individuals who presented as men but identified as women, women who identified as men, and everything in between. It took countless photographs before we managed to guess even a few correctly! It truly ranked among the most bizarre hours I could recall! Still a bit dazed, we broke for lunch, taking a moment to digest both the information and the experience before resuming our training to grasp the medical protocols set by WellPath and the Orleans Justice Center (previously the Orleans Parish Criminal Sheriff's Office, aka OPP, aka Orleans Parish Prison). The following days unfolded with lessons covering infection control, the arrest Intake/Receiving Process Center (IPC—an area where I worked nights post-Hurricane Katrina), navigating inmate sick calls, suicide prevention measures, the medication administration process, addressing immigration housing, guiding drug and alcohol detox, and even coordinating dental appointments. Finally, we tackled the skills checkoff list for new hires.

Chapter 2

Training In The Intake Processing Center

I now find myself reflecting on the journey that has brought me back to this familiar place, nearly full circle since my last chapter here wrapped up in 2009. It all began in 2007 when I ventured into a new dimension of my healthcare career as a Clinical Liaison. This role, pivotal yet often misunderstood, revolves around nursing, but with a unique twist: I would traverse various healthcare facilities—typically stepping into acute care hospitals like the esteemed Ochsner Hospitals in New Orleans—to conduct comprehensive assessments of patients poised to transition to what is called "post-acute" care settings. These include Long-term Acute Care Hospitals (LTACs), Skilled Nursing Facilities (SNFs), Inpatient Rehabilitation Hospitals (IRHs), and a range of others. At that juncture, I was also navigating the turbulent waters of a divorce, coinciding with a recruitment call from a lifelong friend who was convinced that this path would be a good fit for me. Thus, I embarked on the arduous yet rewarding process of becoming a Clinical Liaison. At that time, I felt the weight of burnout pressing heavily upon me, a residue of years spent in correctional healthcare. Now, fast forward 16 years and here I stand, returning to the roots of my career, yet propelled by entirely different motivations and a wealth of experiences that have reshaped my perspective.

Imagine stepping into the intake process of today's justice system—a far cry from the chaos of 2009. Back then, after Hurricane Katrina razed the original facility, we worked in a repurposed food warehouse, grappling with makeshift operations in the wake of devastation. Fast forward to now, and I find myself in a building that feels almost sleek and efficient—a far cry from the memories of flood and ruin. The intake area sprawls impressively, easily accommodating around a hundred seats, flanked by several medical screening stations and a couple of large, flickering televisions. The expansive booking and screening zones contrast sharply with the cramped conditions of yesteryear, as do the numerous holding cells that now seem more humane. As I dive into learning the upgraded computer system and the intricate medical intake process, it's striking just how much the experience has evolved! Though the familiar method of assigning an arrest/folder number to new inmates clings persistently to the past, the medical screening now boasts a level of detail that was unimaginable back then.

The first thing that captured my attention was the vividly colorful "WITHDRAWAL PROTOCOL CROSSWALK" informational sheet plastered on the wall beside the computer. The alarming surge of the drug epidemic and escalating crime rates fueled my desire to write this book. And right here, before me, lay the very framework I needed to plunge into this harrowing subject. COWS and CIWA... What are those, you might wonder? Well, let me unravel that for you.

The Clinical Opiate Withdrawal Scale, commonly referred to as COWS, is a medically administered instrument utilized by clinicians to evaluate the severity of 11 prevalent opiate withdrawal symptoms. This total score derived from these items serves to assess an individual, such as a new arrestee, in terms of their opiate withdrawal level and to determine their physical dependence on opioids. Given the alarming rise in opioid prescriptions for pain management, the accessibility of sublingual buprenorphine—a synthetic opioid designed to alleviate withdrawal symptoms—has markedly increased. So, what exactly is buprenorphine?

Buprenorphine stands as the pioneering medication for treating opioid use disorder, or "OUD." It's a unique option that can be prescribed in various settings, including physician offices, substance abuse treatment centers, as well as jails and prisons. Like all medications involved in treatment, buprenorphine should be a part of a thorough treatment approach that encompasses counseling and additional services, effectively addressing the whole person involved. This principle holds equally true in correctional environments. Curiously enough, the slang names used on the streets for these substances can be quite amusing, and I find them both funny and intriguing. I'm inclined to think you might find them equally entertaining!

So… I'll start with the short-acting opioids and go through each one and tell you their street names. I'll space them out in case you ever want to refer to them. Vicodin (Hydrocodone) has many street names like… and these are from the Withdrawal Protocol form…

- Hydros
- Tabs
- Vikes
- Vitamins
- Bananas (this one made me laugh)
- Dro's and
- Fluff.

Next, we have Oxycontin/Percocet (Oxycodone):

- Hillbilly Heroin
- Oxy
- Ozone
- Roxy
- Berries
- Blues and
- Blueberries… Can't make this shit up lol!

Next, we have Codeine. These are interesting…

- Captain Cody or Cody
- Little C
- Schoolboy (tried to ask around to see why it's called that but couldn't get a definitive answer…) and
- Purple Drank

Okay this next one has roughly seven names, but these are the most common for Heroin:

- Black Tar/Pearl
- Brown Sugar
- China White
- Dradon
- "H"
- Horse and
- Skunk (Heroin + Cocaine = Speedball). I must admit I've heard the term Speedball before but didn't know that it was a combination of the two. Sounds dangerous to me!

The last one of the Short Acting Opioids is Ultram (Tramadol):

- Chill Pills
- Trammies (not to be confused with trannies) and
- Ultras

Settle in because we are just getting started lol.

Next, we have the Long-Acting Opioids. These are interesting as a couple of these are used to help a person in the withdrawal process and one is considered the most lethal and powerful one on the streets.

Methadose (Methadone). An older school withdrawal drug by today's standards but still abused on the streets:

- Dollies
- Dolls
- Amidone
- Fizzies
- Mud (interesting)
- Red Rock and my favorite so far-
- Tootsie Roll

Next, we have Suboxone/Subutex (Buprenorphone):

- Big Whites
- Buse
- Small Whites
- Sobos
- Oranges
- Stops and
- Strips

Next, we have the most well-known drug in the past few years and that is FENTANYL… The killer…

- Apache
- China Girl
- Dance Fever
- Friend
- Goodfella (this one was interesting as Goodfellas is one of my favorite movies ever!)
- Jackpot
- Murder 8
- Tango and Cash

I'm sure there are others, but these are the most common. This wraps up the COWS portion. Next, is the CIWA.

Alcohol…. Self-explanatory but will throw it in there for fun:

- Beer, liquor, wine, spirits and moonshine-Street name:
    - Booze
    - Pruno (can say I haven't heard that one before)

Now on to the Benzodiazepines.

- Diazepam (Valium). Street names:
    - Eggs
    - Jellies
    - Vallies
- Lorazepam (Ativan) and Chlordiazepoxide (Librium) have the same names…
    - Candy
    - Downers
    - Tranks

- Clonazepam (Klonopin)
    - "K"
    - K-Pin
    - Super Valium
- Alprazolam (Xanax)
    - Bars
    - French Fries (really?)
    - Xan

So, if you hear any of these strange names you will know what they are talking about. Last but certainly not least are the Synthetic and other Drugs.

Let's start with Hallucinogens and Psychedelics…

- Mushrooms. Street names:
    - Alice
    - Boomers
    - Shrooms
- PCP. Street names:
    - Angel Dust
    - Purple Rain(lol)
    - Stardust
- Peyote. Street names:
    - Cactus
    - Black Button
    - Green Button
    - Shaman
- Ketamine. Street names:
    - Cat Valium
    - Special K
    - Blind Squid
    - Kit Kat
    - Vitamin K

- LSD. Street name:
    - Acid
    - Dots
    - Sugar Cubes
    - Yellow Sunshine
- Synthetic Cannabinoids. Street names:
    - Spice
    - K2
    - Bath Salts
    - Black Mamba
    - Flakka

Next. Inhalants.

- Nitrous Oxide. Street names:
    - Buzz Bomb
    - Hippe Crack(lol)
    - Laughing Gas
    - Whippets.

Now on to Stimulants…

- Cocaine. Street names:
    - Nose Candy
    - Coke
    - Eight Ball
    - Dice
    - Garbage
    - Grit
    - Devil's Dandruff
    - Crack
- Methamphetamine (Crystal Meth). Street names:
    - Crank
    - Crystal

- Meth Ice
- No Doze (that one's kinda funny)
- Rocket Fuel

- MDMA (Ecstasy)
  - Molly
  - Adam
  - Beans
  - Candy
  - Clarity
  - Dancing Shoes
  - Disco Biscuit (my favorite lol)
  - "E"
  - E-Bomb
  - Egg Rolls.

Well, that concludes just about any way an individual can get high and what they are called on the streets! Moving on...

The Clinical Institute Withdrawal Assessment for Alcohol, commonly known as "CIWA," stands as the predominant approach for addressing alcohol withdrawal, widely embraced by healthcare professionals. While numerous rating scales for alcohol withdrawal exist, the CIWA framework, particularly in its use of benzodiazepines for managing withdrawal symptoms, is thoroughly recognized. Dosing of benzodiazepines that is triggered by symptoms has been shown to result in a reduced treatment duration and less overall medication use compared to a fixed schedule approach. Though initially validated in medically stable patients undergoing alcohol detoxification, the CIWA protocol has extended its application, finding utility in hospitals, jails, prisons, and various detoxification facilities.

This wasn't yet termed "CIWA" or "COWS," and the opioid crisis had not reached its current depths when I embarked on my journey in 2003. At that time, any individual apprehended and deemed likely to undergo withdrawal was directed to HOD-10 (House of Detention), where acute psychiatric patients were housed alongside those requiring monitoring for alcohol or drug detox. Encounters with heavy opioid users were rare; the overwhelming majority of arrestees were grappling with alcohol. What exactly is alcohol withdrawal, you wonder? It encompasses the psychological and physiological turmoil that emerges following a cessation of extended, heavy alcohol consumption. When one abruptly halts drinking, the body suddenly misses the effects of alcohol and must recalibrate to operate without it. The severity of withdrawal symptoms can vary dramatically, hinging on the duration and quantity of alcohol intake. Before Hurricane Katrina, the detox prison tiers of HOD-10 typically housed around 15 to 20 male and female arrestees at any given time. Nowadays, those in need of detox can be found scattered across floors 1, 2, or even 3. It's not the most streamlined approach, but the configuration of the new facilities diverges significantly from what was established before.

In the year 2023, the procedure following an arrest has become remarkably systematic. Upon arrival, the detainee is met with a stringent screening process at the entrance. A medical intake nurse is promptly alerted and makes their way to the door, where the arrestee stands alongside the officers responsible for their detainment. This individual is subjected to a series of pointed questions, designed to assess their medical stability prior to incarceration. Sometimes, they arrive clutching hospital paperwork, evidence of an injury sustained during the arrest, or a pre-existing condition voiced during the encounter. Among these are pregnant individuals battling addiction, brittle diabetics, and others grappling with various health issues. In today's world, a significant number of those apprehended are under the influence of substances, necessitating a thorough medical screening. They face inquiries that reflect an unsettling reality about where society currently stands.

- Have you recently had any drugs or alcohol? If yes, when? What drugs?

This is important as they must be placed on the proper withdrawal protocol with most needing both COWS and CIWA!

- Did you swallow any drugs or place any drugs in a BODY CAVITY?

Yes, that's right… Believe it or not, this does happen, and these days and it happens more often than you might imagine.

- Are you homicidal or suicidal?

Many times, when someone is arrested and if they are intoxicated, many express feelings of being suicidal and if they are pissed off can express being homicidal. Back in 2003, all the suicidal or homicidal (mostly suicidal) would be housed on HOD 10 as well. As you might imagine, HOD 10 could be quite entertaining and hectic at the same time with the acute psych, the detoxing, the homicidal and the suicidal all in close proximity. Full moon nights were always interesting lol. Anyways, on to the other questions…

- Have you been bitten by a dog or person? Have you been tasered?

I've seen a couple of dog bites back in the day and one guy came through the booking area after being tasered and he had 2 perfectly round half inch holes where the taser went right on to both chest walls! Ouch!

- Do you have any mental health problems or are you under the care of a mental health professional?

This can be key especially if the person requires psychiatric medications as going without these can lead to many other problems.

- Do you take any medication or have any medical problems?

This may be obvious but it's always good to have the patient on their medications as quickly as possible especially if they are a diabetic as they can have issues quickly…

- Do you have any wounds, open cuts, sores, or injuries that need immediate emergency room care or that occurred during the arrest?

For obvious reasons, this would need to be addressed right then and there and just about all the time the office/officers will bring the arrested to the hospital on the front end to be medically cleared but everyone involved has to CYA (Cover Your Ass) at that time!

- Do you have any disabilities or known illnesses that may be deemed contagious to others?

I've spoken to some people within the system and as you might imagine, the Covid pandemic wreaked havoc throughout the New Orleans Parish Prison just as it did across the country and presented numerous medical challenges. Thank God I wasn't around to see that but had my own healthcare worker challenges. See the next question.

- Have you recently been exposed to COVID or the Flu and have any symptoms? Are you currently vaccinated against either? This question would be asked a million times, I'm sure and it will be with us all forever it appears.

There are a couple of other screening questions, but these are the main ones.

As I navigate the demands of the day, we've already had a few individuals apprehended, necessitating the detox procedure. Back in 2003, following Hurricane Katrina, the jail saw over fifty arrests daily, whereas now we're averaging between eight to fifteen. The protocols for screening have evolved considerably. Previously, vital signs were assessed at the entrance before one was escorted in. Anyone presenting out-of-range vitals would be promptly dispatched to the hospital for medical clearance. In contrast, the current procedure focuses on ensuring that individuals aren't injured; if they are, the police reroute them to the hospital prior to their time in jail. In those earlier days, if someone was overly intoxicated or precarious, they had to be medically cleared by a hospital before any arrest could proceed.

Just as it had been on my first day back in 2003, I found myself thrust into a storm of chaos. A man was taken into custody after he had gone to the home of his children and their mother—who, regrettably, wasn't there at the time—and set the place on fire, leading to the heartbreaking deaths of those innocent kids. It was a nightmarish scene… They captured him on a nearby surveillance camera, running away as the flames consumed the house… It was utterly devastating. News quickly circulated through the jail about this man's arrest, and little did I know, I would soon have to face this monster, asking him about any medical concerns he might have. Good grief… As he was escorted to the medical screening area, deputies clustered around, eager to catch a glimpse of him. Describing the screening as uncomfortable would be a vast understatement.

Chapter 3

IPC versus THE REST OF THE SYSTEM

After that unsettling reintroduction to IPC, marked by a tragic arrest, the day returned to its usual rhythm. As the shift began to draw to a close, it was time to reach out to the doctor for the necessary physician orders concerning the inmates who had been taken in that day. Following protocol, we were to contact the MD regarding multiple patients—yes, patients, despite the circumstances—at the shift's end, unless someone was experiencing an acute episode or their vital signs indicated they needed immediate attention. Many of the individuals arrested for drug use or intoxication typically displayed symptoms of withdrawal either upon their arrest or shortly thereafter. My training nurse initiated a call to the on-call Nurse Practitioner. However, it wasn't long before tension filled the air; a disagreement erupted over the phone, voices rising in an escalating exchange! A verbal clash ensued, abruptly ended by the other party. The nurse was visibly frustrated. Having been away from this environment for some time, I found myself caught off guard, though not entirely surprised. Moments later, the nurse called back, and with cooler heads prevailing, the orders were finally secured. On my first day back, I confidently volunteered to deliver the charts to the second-floor clinic, where I would be spending the next few hours of my orientation.

It was time for the shift change, and as I stepped into the clinic, I handed over the chart information to the charge nurse, who was already engaged in a heated phone conversation with the IPC nurse. I could hear raised voices, tension in the air, and the charge nurse's frustration was visible. Apparently, there had been an arrestee in the early hours of the morning who had been sent up to the 3rd floor without being placed on the COWS detox protocol, and he was now sporting a dangerously high blood pressure that demanded immediate action. The charge nurse voiced her displeasure, exclaiming that such oversights occurred "far too often…!" I then found a spot to observe as the nurses relayed the day's events to the incoming team for the night shift. The nurse sitting to my right began her report with a grim tone, noting, "Inmate 'A' got jumped today, leaving him with multiple facial lacerations and an orbital fracture… He was sent to University Hospital around 15:30." The following nurse was the Detox nurse, and I leaned in closer, eager to catch her update. She started with another nurse, "We currently have 18 inmates on COWS/CIWA… Inmate 'Z's' blood pressure just hit 172/105… physician notified… Inmate 'D' seized around 14:30 and was routed to University Hospital for further evaluation…" Curious about their detox numbers, I inquired how many were typically under treatment, and she explained it usually hovered between 15 and 25 at any given time. Back in 2003, we managed anywhere from 10 to 20, but they were confined to a single floor (HOD-10). Now, inmates could be spread across the 1st, 2nd, or 3rd floors. It was a stark departure from my experience at HOD-10, but given the differences in facility design, it seemed this was the new necessary approach.

As the day drew to a close, I absorbed the layout of the facility, familiarizing myself with the various floors and the unique units housing the inmates. Rather than cataloging each floor, I'll sketch a broad overview of their purposes. There's a psychiatric tier accommodating those deemed higher risk, alongside a step-down unit for individuals who have stabilized somewhat, managing their mental health largely through medication. Inmates can be placed on suicide watch, a situation taken with the utmost seriousness and subject to constant scrutiny. It's disheartening to witness the reasons why many land in these walls; a sense of despair often hangs heavy in the air upon arrest. When the medical screening includes questions about suicidal thoughts, some respond affirmatively, triggering a process that places them in solitary conditions, garbed in a sleeveless smock, closely monitored, their vital signs taken and probing questions posed throughout the day. On adjacent tiers, there are those in protective custody, higher security, young inmates engaged in schooling, and the so-called "HOLE," where troublemakers are isolated until they're considered fit to mingle with the general population again. The rest of the system includes general population, female psychiatric units, female general population, detox areas, and attempts to group specific medical needs together, such as diabetic inmates, though this isn't always successful. This portion of the facility starkly contrasts with the IPC (Intake Processing Center)! All things considered, it was a comprehensive first day of orientation.

The following day unfolded into yet another long stint at IPC, immersed in learning the intricate medical screening process, reaching out to the doctor for directives, and keenly observing the workflow. Typically, 10 to 20 individuals find themselves arrested within a single 24-hour window—remarkably fewer than in years past—and the current medical assessments are notably more thorough. Increasingly, individuals arrive with a variety of ailments, both physical and, crucially, mental. As society progresses, a significant segment of this population grapples with various psychiatric challenges, over half exhibiting some medical issues or a background steeped in alcohol or drug use, which intrigued me most. Witnessing these individuals being brought in for medical evaluation alongside their booked offenses, I noted the juxtaposition of seasoned deputies and high-ranking officials engaging with their younger counterparts. The atmosphere pulsated with a distinct energy, and occasionally a familiar face would light up in surprise upon seeing me… "G… what's up?! You back?!?!..." Their reactions, often humorous, especially when they learned my connection to Hurricane Katrina, prompted eager inquiries for stories of that tumultuous time. As my orientation progressed from IPC to the tiers, I keenly focused on grasping the daily responsibilities assigned to the nursing staff.

During the day shift, from 7 a.m. to 7 p.m., the RNs took on the crucial responsibility of meticulously reviewing Detox protocol reports alongside any outstanding MD orders, History and Physicals (H&P), and Intake screenings. They also had to keep the ER route logs updated and compile the shift reports, among a myriad of other responsibilities. Meanwhile, the LPNs prepared for the important 8 a.m. Medication Pass, restocked the medication cart, and conducted Detox assessments at 10 a.m. and 2 p.m. Additionally, they evaluated Sick Calls, treated as necessary, and referred patients to medical providers when warranted. They reviewed pending orders, transcribed them, conducted suicide watch evaluations, and managed wound care, i.e., their own extensive list of duties. However, this division of labor appeared to create an imbalance, especially as it became evident that certain tiers were increasingly populated compared to others, causing visible tension amongst the nursing staff. During my stay, I observed both the day and night shift nurses typically remained tethered to their specific tiers. Yet, I quickly noted frequent call-offs and the urgent demands posed by substantial medication passes that loomed on the horizon. Nurses "pulled" from their regular rotations to cover additional duties often found themselves overwhelmed by the sheer volume of medications needing distribution. Witnessing this hectic dance firsthand, it was obvious that this persistent issue was not easily solvable. With a couple of the floors housing over 200 inmates, all requiring medication, the complexity multiplied significantly: nurses needed to pull, pre-pack, and distribute medications across multiple tiers while also performing crucial tasks like checking blood sugars, administering insulin, monitoring blood pressures, and executing other medical procedures—all within a pressing timeframe. This overwhelming orchestration became even more daunting the moment a scheduled nurse called off just before the shift was set to begin.

I was swiftly plunged into the chaos of orientation, thrust into the whirlwind of medication passes. My role as a PRN nurse felt like an initiation rite into this demanding world! In those first few weeks, at least one nurse would call off—one night, a staggering four did! I found myself not only passing the meds but also assisting another late-arriving PRN nurse, scrambling to manage the med pass on a different floor. We toiled until the clock struck 2:30 a.m., and I still had to return to my day job the following morning! I was initially meant to clock out by 11:30 p.m. But hey, I'd much rather face the reality of this tumultuous journey ahead than remain in the dark about what was to come.

This is the crux of the IPC's conflict with the broader system. Throughout numerous medication passes, an inmate will declare that they haven't received their blood pressure medication, all while detoxing from opioids and struggling with high blood sugar levels. They may have told the intake nurse there are no medical issues at hand—cliché excuses like that. When an inmate claims, "I haven't taken my meds in days…" they get shuffled off to the Medical Observation Unit for a full vital signs assessment. More often than not, in this scenario, the inmate was meant to be on a hypertension protocol, with medications prescribed and scheduled for a doctor's visit the very next day. If this oversight comes to light, the night shift nurse manager typically blows a gasket, assuming it's a blunder from the intake team—and it very well could be. Yet, it's just as likely that the inmate misled the intake nurse during the initial process. There are myriad other issues that occur, but this situation remains the most frequent and readily ignites frustration on both sides.

After several nights and intensive training during the days, I was officially on board, taking on shifts, handling medication passes, screening newly arrived arrestees, conducting detox rounds, and filling in wherever necessary. By mid-October 2023, we had just entered flu season. On my second or third shift, I was assigned the detox rotation, tasked with offering flu shots to any inmate, whether male or female, who consented. An infectious disease logbook was meticulously kept to document who received the shot and who opted out. I moved from tier to tier, checking vital signs and applying the COWS and CIWA protocols whenever a detoxing inmate required assistance. It was a far cry from 2003, when everyone was congregated on one floor with a simple detox protocol. Now, it was far more intricate. As I was assessing one female inmate, she suddenly exhibited seizure-like activity; a code was sounded, and the inmate was stabilized, drawing a wide-eyed crowd of curious female inmates! Just like the good old days, but now I was facing a new generation of criminals grappling with even more intense substance abuse issues.

When I first navigated through the maze of orientation, every new arrestee had a checklist that included a TB shot, HIV screening, and a handful of other health checks. They had just started to roll out flu shots during these screenings, but as October dawned, the staff decided it was essential to offer flu shots to everyone in the prison—and track it meticulously. Initially, the process felt like a chaotic scramble, with inmates repeatedly being asked to sign refusal forms over and over in that month. But after some time, the administration worked out the kinks. I began coming in a few times a week from my day job, and without fail, I found myself engulfed in the flu shot rotation—surprisingly entertaining, I must say. Watching these "tough guys" who otherwise exuded bravado, suddenly turn into nervous wrecks at the sight of a needle was a spectacle! Witnessing them squirm while getting the shot, their bravado wavering, was quite the hilarious contrast. There seemed to be no logic behind who opted for the shot and who turned it down. Often, they'd refuse or simply not be offered one during their initial screening, only to change their minds once they settled into their tier or cell.

One night, entirely without warning, nearly everyone on the tier opted for the shot. As soon as they witnessed the first few brave souls line up, the rest quickly followed suit. Personally, I haven't had a flu shot in a decade; it just isn't my thing. But that night was different—maybe it was the magic of the moon or some unseen force at play because I'd estimate that about 30 out of 35 people gave in! It felt almost surreal. I headed over to the adjacent tier where, in stark contrast, not a single one of around 50 individuals took the shot, yet each had to sign a refusal form. It's a bizarre system; they didn't need it, but had to be offered it regardless. This peculiar routine lasted until the new year, turning into my unofficial nightly duty. Eventually, I became the go-to person for administering these shots, embracing the oddities that came with it. Some nights were entertaining, filled with amusing encounters amidst the chaos of fights or detox struggles that permeated the atmosphere. In a strange way, it brought an odd sense of fun, a reminder that each night brought its own surprises, where unpredictability reigned supreme.

Chapter 4

1 Job, Then 2 Jobs, Then 3 Jobs

As I stepped back into the world of nursing, a realm I had first entered two decades prior, I recalled my recent return to Home Health visits and the marketing duties I had taken on for a regional healthcare company in the vibrant city of New Orleans. It had been a significant stretch of time since I had performed venipunctures, IV therapy, injections, and the myriad tasks that make up traditional nursing care. My title, Clinical Liaison, encompassed a blend of marketing and assessing patients for various "post-acute" facilities—a role that felt both familiar and foreign. As I embarked on this intriguing social experiment of returning to work at the prison, it felt like a wise decision to adopt this "day job," granting me the flexibility to continue my evening endeavors. While diving back into this facet of healthcare wasn't my primary desire, I understood the need to adapt and do what was necessary.

Shortly after completing orientation with the home health agency, I was on the brink of embarking on my first patient visits at their residences. This was an entirely new frontier for me, and I must say, it left me both astonished and astounded! My initial visits took me deep into the heart of New Orleans, into neighborhoods most would avoid, yet I found a strange thrill in the challenge. Apparently, I have a penchant for adrenaline, which I can't help but chuckle at. My very first appointment led me to an apartment in the historic 9th ward, a place etched in the shadows of Hurricane Katrina. It was a revelation! Driving through the area, remnants of the destruction still loomed large—ruined buildings and homes stood as somber reminders that the disaster's aftermath felt as if it had just unfolded yesterday.

As I cruised to a halt outside the apartment complex, my eyes fell on a couple of sketchy figures loitering on the corner, their shadows casting unease. Growing up in New Orleans, I learned an invaluable lesson: fear is like a magnet for trouble; but if you project confidence, trouble tends to fade into the background. Yet here we are in 2023, a different landscape unfolding before me, where carjackings and crime rates have soared—a truth I've witnessed firsthand during my evenings at the jail. Shaking off the weight of those thoughts, I hopped out of my car and strolled down the dim corridor to knock on the apartment door. "Come in…" The invitation was casual but carried an air of mystery; I hesitated, then pushed it open. Inside, the patient lounged on his couch, a beer cradled in one hand and a cigarette dangling from the other—classic New Orleans style at 11:00 AM. Surprised? A little, but in this city, nothing's too shocking. As I began my routine questions and took his vital signs, I asked him the reason for his hospital stay, fully aware of the answer but eager to hear his side of the story.

"Well… there I was, caught in the chaos after a car accident with my brother, who had taken flight from the cops when his lights went flashing. He was well aware that a warrant for his arrest loomed over him like a dark cloud, and in his panic, he bolted with me gripped in the passenger seat!" I skimmed over the notes: MVA – Motor Vehicle Accident, followed by MI (myocardial infarct), and

I must admit, this twist caught me completely off guard! My initial thought had been that he suffered a heart attack while behind the wheel, not a calamity during a reckless dash with his sibling away from law enforcement! Incredible!!! Anyway, this guy was undoubtedly a character, and what a wild introduction for my first visit! After wrapping up the consultation, I set off toward my next appointment, off Napoleon Ave in the vibrant heart of Uptown New Orleans.

Whoa! In the blink of an eye, I leaped from the streets to a sprawling mansion! This place was out of this world! Don't get me wrong, I've got some affluent buddies living Uptown, but this estate was on a whole other level! I gave the door a solid knock, and it felt like an eternity before someone appeared. It wasn't the guest I expected, but the maid who welcomed me in and led me to the elegantly furnished living area where the patient lounged in her plush robe. "Hey there…" she greeted, her voice dripping with that irresistible New Orleans charm…

"Good afternoon, ma'am… How are you faring today? I noticed you've just been discharged from the hospital…"

"I certainly have… Would you care for a drink?"

At this juncture, I graciously declined and moved on to check her vital signs, taking a moment to gaze around the expansive living room. For a fleeting second, I considered sharing where I had just been but thought better of it. It was already afternoon, so I continued with a few more visits before diving into paperwork. Soon enough, the hour arrived for my evening shift at the jail. I was still in the data-gathering phase of this social experiment, and each encounter was a fresh chance to observe and document. The evening air felt brisk and cool as I arrived at the facility, where I spotted several units of the NOPD rolling in, officers escorting a handful of arrestees. Tensions were obvious as they began to usher the newcomers into the booking area. Upon entering, the freshly apprehended individuals underwent an initial medical screening to ensure there were no apparent injuries or health issues requiring a trip to the local hospital for clearance before they could be formally processed.

"Man, what the fuck!!!" one of the cuffed individuals belted out…

The cop just looked at me and shrugged his shoulders with an "oh well" look on his face.

After that little outburst, I finally reached the bustling medical clinic in IPC, ready to collect the day's charts and head up to the 2nd floor to begin administering flu shots. It felt like a full moon night as the place buzzed with energy that evening. Hardly five minutes into my shift, a backup call rang out from the 3rd floor tier, where chaos erupted due to multiple altercations—resulting in several unlucky inmates getting pepper-sprayed! And wouldn't you know it, even the deputies fell victim to the pepper spray cloud. If you've never faced that fiery experience, let me tell you, it's a nightmare! Flashback to 2003/2004, when I was stationed on the 10th floor of the HOD building, where a massive fan was used to circulate air during the summer heat—oh, those days were just as wild.

One evening, as I sat enveloped in the sterile glow of the psych clinic while wrestling with paperwork, chaos erupted. Suddenly, two inmates clashed, their shouts slicing through the silence. My gaze snapped up just in time to see two deputies racing down the corridor, urgently brandishing pepper spray as their weapon of choice to quell the situation. Within seconds, the fan whirred ominously, drawing the pungent mist into the air and sending a vile cloud wafting into our small office. The smell was horrendous! Even though we weren't directly hit, my eyes betrayed me, stinging fiercely, and my throat tightened like a vice. It took a solid ten minutes for the burning sensation to dissipate, yet the acrid taste and effects lingered agonizingly for hours. I could hardly fathom what those poor souls must have felt after taking a full blast as they stumbled into medical for treatment.

About eight of them screamed, their faces a mix of fear and pain, the stinging spray eliciting tears from more than just the intensity of the moment. A couple of deputies—both men and women—had unintentionally caught the brunt of it, grimacing through their discomfort. As the chaos began to ebb, I gathered my supplies for the night's flu shots. You might remember the man who was arrested for setting his house ablaze with his children inside, a horrific act that resulted in their deaths. This evening, oddly enough, he was slated for a flu shot. It felt surreal to confront someone so utterly devoid of humanity—an actual cold-blooded killer. His expression was flat, a blank stare that seemed to absorb the light yet reflect none, and my questions were met with a disconcerting silence. Not to mention, he was locked away in maximum-security isolation; I couldn't help but feel a swell of anxiety at the thought of interacting with such evil. Yet, I continually reminded myself of my purpose: to document everything that transpired, no matter how unsettling.

Regardless, he finally agreed to receive the vaccination, signed off on the consent form, and I proceeded with the injection. My mind spiraled into dark thoughts—visions of him facing a future with a lethal injection, not so different from the very one he was receiving now. It's unfathomable to think someone could ignite a fire that takes lives, much less the lives of my own children! The more I contemplated, the more my heart sank, pulling my spirits down with it. It was an overwhelming thought... Just as I wrapped up the procedure, another inmate called out, "Hey doc… I've got a question…" It's a common refrain in my line of work since many assume I'm a doctor—chuckles ensue. I should have been; the pay would've been much nicer.

I spun toward the sound of the voice, only to discover it was echoing from the elevated tier up front. As I made my way closer, another inmate called out, followed by yet another. Frustration bubbled up, and I found myself shouting, "Hold on, fellas… damn…" This was the dreaded "hole," a place reserved for those whose behavior warranted isolation. I understood their desperation for interaction, yet it was annoying. Gratefully, my visits here were infrequent—thankfully, never again, I hoped. The remainder of the night drifted by uneventfully, and by 11:30 p.m., I was ready to collapse into bed. However, just as I neared home, my phone buzzed with a request to cover a shift for a nurse who'd called off, which I politely declined.

The following day greeted me with a weighty agenda, a full slate of patients awaiting my care in their homes. As I made my way to my first appointment, the phone rang, slicing through the morning calm. It was the office, requesting me to divert my path to attend to another patient—one whose caregiver couldn't make it due to sudden illness. It meant I'd have to shuffle my morning schedule around, adjusting the visit times for the other two patients I was slated to see. Lunch? Well, that would just have to be a little later than I'd planned. No worries, just another day in this life.

After collecting all the necessary patient information, I made a call to inform her that I would be visiting today. I arrived around 10:00 a.m., knocking gently on the door, before the patient welcomed me inside to the living room. She resided in a suburb of New Orleans, in a humble house cluttered with boxes, all part of preparations for an impending move. The patient, appearing to be about 65 years old—like many I encountered—had a warmth that eased the initial awkwardness. I always strive to find common ground, especially in a stranger's home, where uncertainty looms.

"Hello there… I'm Gavin… your usual nurse isn't available today, so I'll be taking care of you for this visit…"

The patient was pleasant and appropriate, but, like most first encounters, there was a slight awkwardness to the initial introduction.

"Hello… welcome in…"

Before I stepped in, I briefly read the patient's chart and orders, noting the wound care that was necessary. It struck me as peculiar that the patient was wearing a robe, but as I delved deeper into the specifics of the wound care, the choice of attire began to make some sense.

"Don't be alarmed when you see my wounds… I've had them for a long time and I'm not sure if they will ever heal…" To my surprise, they appeared quite fresh, but they weren't. It was just the nature of the autoimmune disease that the patient had.

"No worries…." I mumbled, and I began to remove some of the bandages that were covering the larger wounds.

These wounds were, without a doubt, the most excruciating-looking I had ever encountered on a patient. My heart sank at the thought of removing them, praying that the process wouldn't involve too much pain for the individual. It was clear that the patient had endured countless wound care treatments before, so I carried out the procedure while keeping the patient's comfort in mind.

About halfway through our conversation, we wandered into various topics, including my father's past as a jazz musician. I casually mentioned I was working part-time at the prison. To my astonishment, the patient instantly replied, "I spent years there as a psychiatrist before Hurricane Katrina…" My jaw dropped! What were the chances? Amazingly, I said, "No way!! I joined in 2003, stayed through Katrina, and worked part-time until 2009… I recently returned…"

From there, an engaging conversation unfolded. We explored a myriad of topics, exchanging vivid tales of our experiences amidst the trials we faced. When she discovered I had penned a book chronicling my father and me enduring the harsh reality of being stranded, her curiosity was piqued, and she expressed a keen interest in diving into my story.

"Wow… sounds fascinating! Can't wait to read it! How is your dad these days…"

I let the patient know he passed away in November of 2014 and of course, condolences were given.

"Well, thank you… He lived a full life, for sure!"

After a few more minutes of conversation, I informed the patient that I needed to attend to a few others and eagerly anticipated our next discussion. The patient expressed gratitude for my assistance with the wound care and our exchange about the prison. As I drove away, I remained in a state of disbelief that, among all the patients I could have encountered, I had met one who worked at the very facility where I was undercover and bore firsthand knowledge of life there. I generally scoff at coincidences, and at that moment, it struck me that God was unmistakably stepping in, presenting me with this task to fulfill. There was no doubt about it.

On that note, to my astonishment, just a few weeks later, another patient was added to my rotation, who resided in the gritty depths of New Orleans East. As I approached their home for our first meeting, an odd sense of recognition washed over me upon seeing them. The moment I stepped inside, my eyes were drawn to the walls, which were adorned with photographs showcasing this individual alongside various notable New Orleans figures, as well as a collection of vintage boxers capturing the spirit of bygone days. Engaging in conversation, I noticed some poignant Katrina memorabilia displayed prominently, and suddenly, it all clicked. This person was none other than a former high-ranking official from the legacy of Orleans Parish Prison. I was astounded! Another unexpected link to my past... Absolutely wild.

We chatted about the current facility and regime, discussing how it is now compared to back then, and the patient was fully aware but didn't have much good to say...

"Hard to believe... the shit goin' on there would have never happened on my watch..."

I agreed...

After that encounter with the other patient tied to the "system," I found myself reflecting on my evening off. A part of me was electrified by the day's revelations, igniting a strong desire to dive back in and unearth more information. Yet, I was acutely aware that fatigue was creeping in; I'd been burning the candle at both ends. The temptation to revisit the past, particularly the insights shared by the new patient, was nearly unbearable. But the old HOD 10 building, a relic that had stood silent for years, was a fortress, locked away from my curiosity. My thoughts raced, filled with questions and possibilities. I knew there would be future opportunities to unravel these mysteries, but tonight, rest had to take precedence.

By this time with the home health, I had seen some interesting cases/patients... Here are a few with some intriguing medical conditions living in some crazy places...

Mid-September... A man in his late forties, blind and battling diabetes, resides in a sprawling, crumbling post-Katrina apartment complex that feels surreal to encounter. Arriving for my first visit, I rolled into the complex, veering to the right, and I began to second-guess my navigation—had I misdialed the address? This part of New Orleans was unfamiliar territory, and apprehension crept in. My instincts whispered that I might have wandered into a troubled neighborhood, informed by the weight of my years spent in the city. The initial sighting was far from promising; the first few structures I passed felt abandoned, with shattered windows boarded up in hasty escapes and graffiti marking their decay. There was a deep-rooted skepticism settling in—this couldn't possibly be right. I continued to cruise slowly, peering into the fading sunlight that highlighted more neglect, until, around the back of the complex, I spotted a solitary figure. A man was navigating his way across the cracked asphalt, propelling himself forward in a wheelchair, making his way to the front. It struck me then: "This can't be real."

I pull up my car in front of the dilapidated "S" building, scanning the surroundings for the elusive "T," my hands busy with a bag, a stethoscope draped around my neck, and my trusty iPad in tow. The area exudes an aura of neglect, but I forge ahead, navigating to the right side of building "S." As I round the corner, my gaze fixes on a sliding glass door, completely obliterated, shards of glass glinting menacingly in the light, some fragments still clinging to the rugged metal frame.

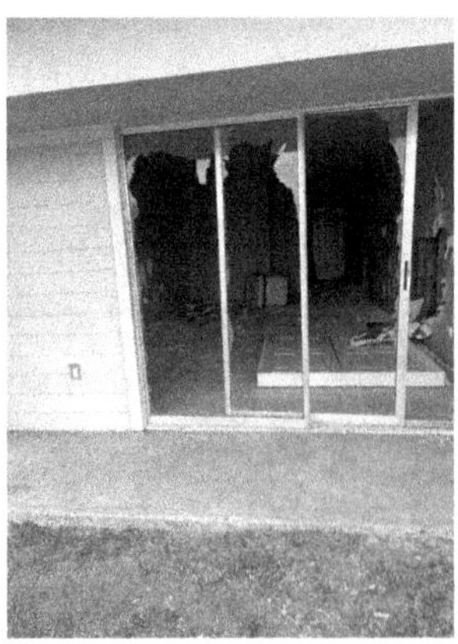

As I venture a bit further down the path, I spot a sign that reads, "Building U," and it dawns on me that I should have turned right instead of left. After a brief search, I finally locate the patient's apartment and give the door a firm knock. A faint voice floats through the air, instructing, "go around to the back..."—a direction that's oddly close to where I'd parked my car. I make my way around, my footsteps echoing softly against the pavement, and I come across a sliding glass door that's ajar, partially concealed by a hanging sheet. "Hello?" I call out, thinking it must be the patient. A raspy female voice responds, "come in..." Hesitating for a moment, I call out the patient's name, and she urges, "come on in... he's in the bathroom."

I ducked beneath the sheet and stepped inside. Wow... This woman appeared, blissfully high and lost in her own world. Just as I was about to utter a word, a small man emerged from what seemed to be a bedroom, his right hand brushing lightly against the wall as he made his way forward. Clearly blind, he paused in the middle of the room and introduced himself with a surprising calmness.

"Hi there... I'm J.B."

I'm going to use initials and "their or them" to protect the privacy of people as I make my way through this adventure.

"Hi Mr. B... I'll be checking you out today..."

We navigated to a small, unkempt table nestled in the corner of the living room. He rummaged through his backpack, claiming his glucose monitor was lurking somewhere beneath. As I conducted his assessment and took his vital signs, a woman lingered nearby, watching intently. At one point, her curiosity got the better of her, and she cheekily asked, "Can you check me out too?" I deftly side-stepped her inquiry, focusing on him. It struck me as amusing that this patient had Ozempic prescribed without having taken it yet. Having seen commercials and knowing friends and family members who were on it, I found it hard to picture him using it. After all, it's pricey and primarily touted for weight loss. I had rarely encountered it prescribed for an average diabetic and couldn't help but wonder if they had decided to prescribe it once weekly due to his blindness.

Anyway, I picked it up and figured out how to use it. It was my first encounter with this type of insulin device, and, let me tell you, I had to go through the instructions—who knew? Its triangular top was quite peculiar, but I managed to get it working and administered the dose. The patient seemed like a genuinely nice guy, and I paused for a moment, trying to picture what it would be like to navigate life in this world without sight. It's a hard life, no doubt. I told him I'd swing by next week to check on him, then made a quick exit before the woman—I wasn't keen on finding out who she was—could ask me to check her vital signs too. I had to bolt!

Navigating my way out of that place was yet another adventure. The apartment complex stretched out before me, its numerous aging buildings bearing the weight of neglect. Situated far from the bustling I-10 interstate, which slices right through the heart of New Orleans, this section, known as "The East," has a reputation for being tough and unruly. Exiting this complex certainly fit that description. Abandoned vehicles littered the landscape, graffiti marred the walls of a few buildings, and overflowing trash dumpsters emitted a pungent odor into the air. Shifty figures lingered around, their postures exuding a sense of wariness. I pressed on, eager to escape, but had to keep my speed in check due to a minefield of potholes and the remnants of old speed bumps. Finally, I emerged onto the I-10, heading back toward downtown—a clear picture of resilience in a challenging neighborhood, yet I stood out as the only blind soul navigating through the shadows of a rough terrain.

Here's another patient/situation that comes to mind: I'll never forget...

I received a call from a colleague the previous day, inquiring if I could take on a few extra patients due to his unfortunate car accident, which had resulted in a fractured neck. Naturally, I was more than willing to assist, so I set about collecting the patients' information. The first step in my routine is always to secure the address and phone number, then reach out to the patient directly. The address rang a bell; it was located in a notoriously unpredictable area of town. Still, my concern was minimal, as I was poised to offer my care.

After several attempts, I still couldn't reach the patient, yet I noted they were due for their monthly psychotropic injection. Nothing to worry about, I thought—at least, that was my initial assumption. I had administered these injections before, but this time would be different, as it would occur in a home environment. Since I couldn't connect with the patient, I decided to place them at the end of my busy schedule on this particular day. As the hours ticked by, my day unfolded much like any ordinary day until I made my way to the patient's residence. However, the neighborhood seemed to deteriorate with each passing block. My instincts were keen, and I felt a heightened sense of awareness, my senses primed for whatever awaited me ahead.

As I arrived at the destination, I noticed it sat at the corner, enclosed by a wrought iron gate that guarded a modest 4-plex, its upper and lower apartments in New Orleans' uptown and mid-city. With my bag in hand, I approached the gate, which sported a weathered "Beware of Dog" sign—a common sight in these parts. Not eager to tempt fate by opening the gate, I decided to sidestep caution. Making my way around to the side, I caught sight of a few individuals lounging casually nearby, their laughter mingling with the vibrant atmosphere. "Hey... I am looking for Mr. H.S..."

I think I startled them a little, as one of them blurted out in an aggressive manner, "Who's there?!?!"

My antenna was up already, and now my adrenaline was starting to flow.

“I'm here to see H.S. to give him his shot..."

Another voice chimed in "ok I'm here... Come around to the other gate, and I'll let you in."

As I approached the front door, I spotted three dubious figures—one leaning casually, while the other two lounged at a patio table, their eyes sizing me up with thinly veiled suspicion. They definitely had the vibe of “tweakers,” and the patient didn’t look much better, disheveled and fidgety. When I stepped inside, disbelief washed over me. Not that I had any prior experience, but I was certain this must be a “crack house!” Chaos reigned; junk was strewn about, the air thick with neglect. The patient beckoned me toward the kitchen, collapsing in a chair while I opted to remain standing. Mere moments passed before he began to ask for a few bucks, his tweaker pals gradually encroaching on the table like scavengers. A feeling of unease crept in… Sure, I had cash on me, but there was no way I was reaching for my wallet with those guys lurking nearby.

“Na man… Don’t travel in the city with any cash (that was a lie, but like I said, my wallet was never coming out of my pocket). Let me go ahead and check your vital signs…”

Between the “crack house” I found myself in and these tweakers, I knew I had to get out of here quickly.

The patient then blurted out, “The last guy that was here giving me my shot gave me a few bucks last time… come on, man… help me out…”

As he spoke, I was steadying my hand, preparing the injection, sweeping my gaze across the room, scanning for the quickest exit. A visceral fear gripped me; the threat of a gun pressed to my skull felt imminent. Keeping my demeanor calm, I said, “Next time, bro… I really can’t help you with that… pull your sleeve up, please, so I can give you this shot…” During this tense moment, I noticed one guy shifting, stepping back, and maneuvering to my left. Uncertainty clouded my mind—what was he up to? In response, I pivoted away, ensuring I kept him in my sights. Swiftly, I plunged the needle into the patient's upper right arm, injecting the medicine, then yanked the needle free, discarding it into the red sharps container nestled by my bag. Just then, another guy pulled up a chair, inching closer to the patient. My heart raced as I gathered my belongings, an instinctual certainty coursing through me: soon, I'd either be robbed or shot right there. It was a feeling I'd never encountered before, and one I hoped to evade forever…

"Alright sir… you're good to go… I'll be sure to tell the other nurse that I saw you, and maybe he will have some cash for you next time..." I was panicking a little, but I was certain I was about to potentially die right here!

I could see the surprise in the patient's eyes, and he reacted about how I would have expected.

"Hey man... What's your hurry..."

I knew they knew I was onto them, and I could see them freeze up a little. I got the feeling they were going to try something, and they knew I knew what they were thinking about doing.

"Yeah man I've got a couple of other patients to see today and have to get going..."

I could see a couple of the tweakers start to back up from their chairs as I just continued to pack my stuff up. I heard the faint sound of a police car's siren in the distance, and they seemed to hear it too as I picked my bag up and made my way to the front door.

"Hey man... Your vital signs are good... Your usual nurse will be back next time... Hopefully, he's recovered from the car accident he was in and be sure to let the home health know if you have any issues that need attention..."

By this point, I was telling him this as I walked to the front door, not trying to come across as worried about the situation. I wasn't sure, but I got the feeling whatever they were contemplating doing wasn't going to happen. Divine intervention, I believe... It wasn't my time, I guess...

I got to my car quickly and drove off, pretty much in a bit of shock! Ironically, the next day, I had to see a patient who lived less than a mile from where that patient lived, near historic St Charles Avenue, in a big ol' nice house. Like I said before, New Orleans is quite unique in that respect.

A few weeks slip by, and I find myself reconnecting with my new patient, observing her insights into what we discussed the last time I saw her. I handed her a copy of my original book, eager to hear her thoughts. Meanwhile, I have taken on another patient located in the 7th Ward of New Orleans, nestled in what is often referred to as the Bywater area. This part of town is a mix of charm and menace, with certain blocks exuding warmth while others evoke genuine trepidation. On this occasion, I received a report from a colleague who had admitted a patient the previous day; the admission took place in the patient's son's car, which deviates from our usual procedure of checking the home environment for any potential trip hazards before proceeding. The nurse did mention the neighborhood's less-than-stellar reputation, leaving me unsure about what awaited me. True to form, I reached out to the patient the night before, only to be met with silence. However, I managed to speak with her son, who assured me she would return home post-dialysis, around noon, and that I was welcome to visit afterward. We settled on 1 PM, and after grabbing a quick bite, I set off toward the 7th Ward, anticipation mingling with a hint of unease.

As I navigate through the streets on my maps app, the situation appears to be deteriorating rapidly. I find myself making a hasty U-turn and halting at a cross intersection, the red light glaring, with two vehicles idling in front of me. My gaze drifts to the left, where a figure leans inside an open car window, while another occupant lounges in the back seat, both engaged in a hushed exchange. A sense of unease washes over me; something feels off-kilter. Suddenly, the driver's side door swings open, and a shifty-looking guy emerges, scanning the surroundings with an intensity that raises my awareness. Meanwhile, the red light persists, and I'm swiveling my head, acutely aware that this could be the silent orchestration of a drug deal unfolding before me. As the light shifts to green, I notice the car in front is still stationary. On this one-way street, passing is a non-option, trapping me in this moment of tension. After a short eternity of three seconds, I slam my palm on the horn, the sound slicing through the air. The character leaning in jolts upright, startled, and makes a hasty retreat across the street, disappearing around the corner like a person caught in the act. Finally, the lead car begins to move as I lock eyes with the guy stepping out of the car as I drive past—a moment heavy with tension.

In my side mirror, our gaze met again, amplifying the adrenaline that surged through me. My heart was pounding as I navigated the intersection, acutely aware that any second could bring danger if I dared to look away. I needed to be ready for anything. After turning toward the patient's house, I inhaled deeply, striving to regain my composure. The address was only a couple of blocks away, but I sensed trouble looming. I parked briefly, scanning my surroundings like a hawk, before inching toward the designated location. As I approached, a knot tightened in my stomach; four cars were stationed in front of the house, and a group of 5 to 7 people lounged around, seeming to stretch the boundaries of normalcy. One individual leaned in a car window, casting suspicious glances. Thirty seconds passed, and the unease grew unbearable—I knew deep down that this was wrong. I slowly drove away, feeling eyes upon me from the porch, their stares sharp and judgmental. Decision made, I steered clear of that scene. Once safe, I called the office and informed the Director of Nursing of the unsettling episode. After some back and forth, she acknowledged the threat and assured me she would notify the doctor's office about the risks involved, leading to the patient's discharge from home health services. With that tense encounter behind me, I wrapped up my day and shifted focus toward the jail, preparing for vital observation and information retrieval.

As I arrived at the facility, I parked my car and looked to turn right at the old HOD building, which triggered some HOD 10th floor memories rushing back like a tide from that life-altering week in August 2005. The space where I had parked my car, nearly identical to where my father and I had once left ours, stood as a silent witness to the floodwaters that swept through, consuming both our vehicles within hours. It's hard to fathom that nineteen years have slipped away since then, and with my father gone nearly a decade, it's astonishing how time blurs the edges of everything…

As I clocked in to administer flu shots, a vivid flashback jolted me to that earlier incident—the drug deal gone awry that could have turned catastrophic. I shook my head, grinning at the absurdity of it all; there I was, just minding my own business, when it felt like my own car had transformed into a target! While I got the report from the day-shift nurse, I recounted the day's earlier drama. Her brow furrowed in shock but also understanding; after all, she hailed from New Orleans and was well acquainted with the chaotic backdrop of that area. Once the report was finished, I learned that a nurse had called off, leaving me to cover the drug and alcohol detox shift until 11:00 PM while squeezing in flu shots when I could. This was ideal since I yearned to delve deeper into the stories of this segment of our inmate population. With the holidays looming, I anticipated a surge in arrests related to drug and alcohol issues. Time would tell if my hunch was correct!

On this evening, I found myself with about an hour to spare before I needed to check on the detox inmates. I figured I'd tackle the flu shots for the diabetic inmates on the fourth floor first. It's well known that diabetics are often more vulnerable to the flu, and let's not forget how that was amplified during COVID—talk about a whole other level of madness, thanks to those lab-created super-viruses. I digress! So, I got to work administering a few shots, but some inmates outright refused, exercising their right to say, "Y'all ain't about to kill me with that nonsense!" or something equally colorful, which made me chuckle. I can't fault them, honestly. I myself haven't had a flu shot in over a decade and have miraculously dodged the flu since. Sure, I believe that the elderly should get vaccinated, given their higher susceptibility, but as for me, I'll pass! I remember a coworker from a few years back who got the flu shot and ended up catching both strains of the flu that season! Talk about brutal! In a place like this, packed into confined spaces, the potential for spreading illness is serious business.

I was chatting with some of the medical staff when I first arrived, curious about their experiences during the COVID crisis. They described it as wild, as you might expect. Inmates and healthcare workers were frequently sent to hospitals, creating a logistical chaos. The hospitals themselves were overwhelmed; no surprise there. During the peak of the pandemic, I served as a Clinical Liaison in New Orleans, tasked with visiting various hospitals to perform bedside evaluations for transfers from Short Term Acute Care Hospitals to Long Term Acute Care Hospitals. LTACHs were established back in the 1980s to ease the patient overflow during times of crisis or something as intense as a PANDEMIC, and oh, did we need them! I won't bore you with the finer points of the healthcare and insurance labyrinth, but many insurance companies are reluctant to approve transfers to LTACHs, always wanting to send patients to a lower level of post-acute care.

The Covid pandemic flipped that situation on its head. The sheer volume of patients filling hospitals in New Orleans and across the globe was unprecedented! Personally, I encountered sights I'd never imagined. Before stepping onto a hospital floor, I had to don an outfit that mirrored a space suit—completely covered, I encountered over a hundred patients, many connected to ten or more IV drips! It was astonishing to witness. Usually, a seriously ill patient would have three or four drips, yet there I was, witnessing eight to ten feeding into individuals in an ICU setting. Fortunately for me, it was two years later during a vacation in New York, with my then-girlfriend and her daughters at an airport, that I finally caught Covid. It was a crowded scene, and upon returning home, I found myself feeling unwell. Thankfully, I only battled mild nasal congestion and body aches—far less severe than what I had observed in the wards. Many of those patients were from nursing homes, which suffered drastically during the pandemic. On average, nursing homes in New Orleans saw a 40% loss of their pre-pandemic population, a heartbreaking statistic. I heard that one nursing home had to keep bodies in a back area since the coroner was unable to move them to the morgue—there simply wasn't enough space…

Anyway, back to the jail… the remainder of the night was consumed with checking vital signs, probing questions, and gathering information. Most of those on the detox protocol found themselves behind bars for either possession or distribution of drugs. The various stages of detox can be, to put it mildly, quite revealing. It's almost easy to spot someone who's been on a long-term substance binge, particularly those who've dabbled with meth; their skin takes on a gray hue, and they typically seem much older than they actually are. Just the day before, I had a home health patient whose appearance spoke volumes about a troubled past with drugs or alcohol, and it wouldn't shock me in the least if our paths crossed again here…

As the weeks rolled into December, Christmas time was upon us. My days were a blend of home health visits and hours spent at the prison, each space resonating with a peculiar kind of irony. Entering homes that were often fractured in spirit, I tried to sprinkle a bit of holiday cheer across their curtains. Some families poured every scarce resource into their decorations, using whatever they could scrounge or piece together to transform their worn spaces into festive havens, while others boasted homes that could rival Macy's flagship in New York! Even the prison had plastered up Christmas decorations; a curious gesture, really, though I pondered how one could truly embrace the holiday spirit behind bars.

Christmas arrived on a Monday in 2023, and I received a call from the scheduling coordinator, inquiring if I could cover a Christmas Eve shift. My initial reaction was hesitance, but curiosity tugged at me; I couldn't help but wonder if there would be a surge in alcohol-related arrests given the festive climate. Family tensions on Christmas Eve? It seemed all but guaranteed—just a hunch, of course. My plan for the evening was to put in some hours in the IPC area, followed by administering flu shots, as I had taken on that responsibility nearly single-handedly. There was a thrill in anticipating an uptick in alcohol and drug-related busts. Domestic violence incidents were also on my radar—unfortunately, a frequent occurrence during the holidays! The night was frosty as I scanned my badge to enter the facility and then made my way to the second-floor body scanner. It's worth mentioning that prior to my return, the facility had seen several overdoses triggered by various circumstances. Apparently, some of the arrested had cleverly hidden drugs in, let's say, less-than-standard body cavities, which led to improper searches during the arrest process, culminating in these overdoses. There were even allegations of deputies smuggling substances in and distributing them to inmates—absurd! The thought of risking my career and freedom to facilitate drug use among inmates was unfathomable. Some deputies had even been arrested for this very crime. Mind-boggling! As a response, strict measures were enforced: no cell phones, no food, nada could get past the entrance without going through rigorous screening.

After successfully navigating the body scanner, I strolled into IPC, where several detainees lounged in the main sitting area. A few were on their phones, making those all-important one-call. I had a strong feeling this night was shaping up to be anything but dull.

I stepped into the medical area and picked up the arrest log for a quick glance. The day was marked by a slightly elevated number of arrests; nothing too wild, yet above the norm. After receiving a few reports on the latest arrestees, I slid into my chair in front of the screening computer, ready to call out the next name for medical evaluation. The guy who approached looked rough around the edges! He bore the unmistakable signs of a chronic drinker or heavy substance user…

"Hey! What's your name, sir…"

I called, only to be met with silence. Either he didn't hear or simply opted not to respond.

"Hey! Yo! What's your name…"

Finally, he responded, his voice weary, either from exhaustion or perhaps the remnants of whatever substances he was on.

"Hey man… It's H.S."

I could sense this screening would be a bit of a challenge, but I was ready for it. After a bit of back and forth with questions and responses, he admitted to being involved in a scuffle at a local bar, just after being kicked out of a rehab facility for the very issues that had landed him in cuffs. Great… Anyway, I wrapped up his assessment and placed him on the detox protocol. An unusual thought struck me at that moment: perhaps I should consider seeking a part-time job at a drug/alcohol rehabilitation facility. It could be insightful to explore the connections between the environments of treatment and incarceration...

A few weeks passed, and suddenly, we found ourselves in the new year. Can you believe it's already 2024? Time has a sneaky way of slipping through our fingers. One evening, after surviving a particularly challenging detox check—where I encountered a twenty-something male transitioning to female, battling a heavy opioid addiction, accentuated by small tattoos adorning the sides of her/his face and striking blue hair—I felt the weight of the world. Clearly, she/he was struggling to find her/his way. After that eye-opening experience, I settled down at a back-office clinic computer, fingers poised to dive into the depths of the internet. My mission? To unearth substance abuse facilities in New Orleans, hoping for a glimmer of opportunity—a part-time nursing job for those elusive weekend or evening shifts. To my astonishment, the city was teeming with facilities, yet the part-time evening jobs were a rarity, a cruel twist in the quest for balance amidst the chaos.

After a relentless search, I finally uncovered a potential gig for a night nurse from 5 p.m. to 11 p.m. Perfect timing… I stepped out of the jail into the biting cold, feeling winter's grip tighten around me. This year's chill was particularly harsh, and tonight was no exception. The prison loomed against the backdrop of I-10, the major thoroughfare that slices through downtown New Orleans. As I hurried to my car to warm it up, the ominous sound of screeching tires erupted from the highway, followed by some sort of crash. Startled, I jumped into my car and made my way toward the on-ramp, where the scene unfolded before me: a vehicle, mangled and toppled onto its side. It was around midnight, and a parade of curious onlookers slowed to gawk at the wreckage, myself included. From my vantage point, I couldn't peer inside, but a few brave souls had already pulled over, darting toward the wreck to assist whoever might be trapped. With a heavy heart, I finally tore myself away and made my way home, exhausted.

The following morning, I tuned into the local news, and mere moments into the broadcast, I heard about a car slipping on black ice along the Interstate just after midnight, flipping multiple times; yet the driver emerged with only minor scrapes! I suppose when fate calls, there's little you can do. After seeing a handful of patients that day, I felt the urge to take a drive and explore a couple of facilities to gauge the neighborhood's vibe. New Orleans is a peculiar patchwork of geography. The mighty Mississippi snakes southward towards the Gulf, but here's the kicker: the West Bank, whimsically dubbed the "best bank" around these parts, lies to the east of downtown, defying all geographical logic. It's a quirky little quirk of this city! The demographics present a curious blend, too. Just a few blocks can transport you from grandeur—glistening mansions—to a stark hood vibe within mere minutes. With New Orleans being ancient compared to Houston or Dallas, it feels like everyone is crammed together here in a basin by a colossal river. Back in the 20th century, New Orleans reigned as one of America's wealthiest cities thanks to its bustling port; yet over time, it has morphed into a tapestry of affluence intertwined with pockets of poverty. Quite a bizarre arrangement, indeed.

I drove past a few different places, taking a good look at what they had to offer before settling on the one that caught my eye for its potential job. It was perfectly aligned with my desired working hours and exactly what I needed to keep my social experiment going. Nestled in the lively core of New Orleans, just a stone's throw from downtown, it seemed like an ideal location for my plan.

The proximity would allow me to easily hop from one job to the next without the hassle of trekking all the way home to Kenner, the suburb where the airport is. That evening, I decided to head back and apply for the position—I couldn't pass up the opportunity to score my third job!

Chapter 5

A Whole New World

As I sit at my desk, the glow of the computer screen illuminating my thoughts, I'm grappling with the logistics of this job application. My evenings are already claimed by the prison, where I only work a handful of shifts each week. Yet, this new opportunity calls for a PRN nurse during the exact hours —5:00 p.m. to 10:00 p.m.—I'm already committed elsewhere. It feels like a riddle with no solution. I pause, weighing my options, and ultimately decide to apply first. Who knows? If I land the job, I'll just have to untangle this schedule later.

A few days passed before the call came in from the facility, inviting me for an interview. To my surprise, it went exceptionally well, and they hired me on the spot, immediately requesting a drug screening at a nearby clinic. It threw me for a loop, but then again, being a substance abuse treatment center, they had their reasons to ensure I wasn't secretly hunting for drugs or had any underlying issues. Fascinating, right? Anyway, after the drug test and formal hiring, my orientation was set for the following Monday. Coincidentally, this happened to be just before Mardi Gras, a time when the city turns into a chaotic whirlwind of festivities, and the jail would undoubtedly be swamped with activity. So, we agreed to push my orientation back another week, which turned out to be a relief. It granted me extra time to strategize my approach while also giving me the chance to witness the wild frenzy of the jail during the Mardi Gras madness.

Well, Mardi Gras 2024 at the jail was quite the spectacle, with numerous arrests for alcohol and drug offenses throughout the weekend and right up until Fat Tuesday. A plethora of colorful characters streamed through, some whisked away on a "fast track" release, while others found themselves stuck in the confines of their cells, spending their festive days behind bars—surprisingly, with a touch of irony, chuckling at their misfortune. To qualify for the coveted fast track, one must either "know" someone in the right position or get bail processed swiftly, without any warrants lurking in their history. It's not every day that you see arrested individuals being expedited through the system, but occasionally, fate smiles—at least, on a select few. Arrests made during the Mardi Gras festivities can bring complications since many essential services—including the courts—simply shut down for the celebrations. With no court in session, the path to bonding out or gaining an outright release becomes steep and treacherous. Nevertheless, amidst all this chaos, one particularly intriguing case captured my attention.

A grandmother, grandfather, and their daughter found themselves in handcuffs, all because of the alleged kidnapping of a grandchild. The background was tangled: the daughter, embroiled in a nasty divorce and fierce custody battle, had seized her child from the father and crossed state lines, seeking refuge at her parents' home in New Orleans. They had lingered there for a spell before the law caught up with them, leading to their untimely arrest. When I first laid eyes on the grandmother, seated in distress, she mirrored the weight of her predicament; her face was a canvas of sorrow and fear, yet she drew strength from the presence of her daughter beside her, despite the fact that it was her daughter's actions that had led them here. What a tangled web they wove. My encounter with her came with the backstory of their ordeal; my role was merely to check her vitals as she underwent a detox protocol. Reports indicated she had been dependent on a daily dose of benzodiazepines prior to her arrest, prompting the need for her to remain medically stable in this dire environment. Once my assessment was finished, I returned to the clinic, eager to relay my observations about the elderly woman to the charge nurse. That's when the full picture unfolded before me. It appeared the grandparents were either oblivious to the seriousness of the situation or simply choosing to ignore it. Regardless, I'd never encountered anything quite like it before, and the truth of what transpired remained elusive, lost as it was on my final day there.

Securing a spot on the Sheriff's office schedule was always a bit tricky, despite their glaring understaffing. They usually reached out to me only during emergencies or when someone was taking a much-needed break since I was PRN, or part-time, at best. Truth be told, their preference leaned heavily toward full-time nurses, but I had no intention of locking myself into that chaotic scene. As the calendar flipped into the New Year of 2024, my duties had dwindled to administering flu shots and offering detox support, which was perfectly fine by me. I had absorbed most of what I needed to learn and had meticulously documented my observations. I planned to keep my name active in their system, just in case any PRN shifts popped up that aligned with my flexible schedule. Honestly, I wasn't losing any sleep over it.

Now, I have this new potential opportunity at the rehab facility to expand my observation of the criminal and social workings of substance abuse. I had a feeling they would be somewhat intertwined, and I would soon find out.

I took a few days off to transition from the confines of the prison system into the realm of rehab. This was uncharted territory for me, so I delved into research on how rehab facilities operate and what I might encounter. The truth was, I should brace myself for an array of bizarre incidents and unpredictable moments, as many of the folks I'd meet were teetering on the brink of a poor choice that could land them back behind bars. My orientation was nothing short of a whirlwind. I was scheduled to work from 5 PM to around 10 PM. Upon arriving and heading up to the second-floor medical clinic, I immediately noticed a growing line of patients eager to snag their 5 PM meds. Inside the clinic, amidst the bustle, I spotted a couple of patients already receiving their prescriptions. A nurse caught my eye, her face lighting up with enthusiasm as she approached.

"What's up, man!" she greeted with infectious energy.

She had a warm vibe, her Rasta-inspired look marked by long, flowing dreadlocks. As I introduced myself, my attention was drawn to a patient behind the counter, who was opening a cabinet door with curious urgency, retrieving a small plastic tub filled with pill bottles. Just then, a nurse handed another patient a set of his own medications from similar bottles. "Yeah, these patients are all adults and can grab their own meds," the nurse explained, a hint of amusement in her tone. I couldn't help but respond, caught off guard, "I hear ya!..."

As I settled in to observe the med pass, each individual who shuffled through the line was undeniably a character in their own right; some exuded a quiet mystery, while others peppered me with questions like,

"Who are you??"

With a grin, I gladly introduced myself, sharing my purpose for being there. The evening unfolded in a whirlwind of learning, taming the computer systems, and mastering the delicate art of entering medications into the electronic medicine registry. With my next day of orientation trailing a few days behind me, I returned for round two only to discover that the nurse who had been my guide was no longer on the scene—fired, just like that! I couldn't fathom the reason, though my intuition hinted it might be linked to what I witnessed during that med pass. Was this the norm? On my inaugural day, certainty had eluded me. The director had mentioned plans to overhaul existing processes, which was part of the rationale behind my hiring. As I grappled with my mounting curiosity, I couldn't help but second-guess my choice to join the team—just kidding!

On this day of orientation, I found myself under the watchful eye of the Clinical Director as she guided me through the meticulous process of inputting medications. These vital substances were sourced from a network of pharmacies affiliated with the facility, necessitating timely entry into the system. Deliveries arrived throughout the week, typically between 2:00 and 5:00 p.m., just as I would be clocking in around 5:00 p.m. It seemed I'd be diving headfirst into the whirlwind of the 5 p.m. med pass, making this a cornerstone of my responsibilities here. Once I navigated that initial deluge, I was also set to embark on an extensive 40 hours of computer training, delving into every aspect of healthcare concerning the substance abuse rehabilitation patient. I learned that this training had to be completed within 30 days to ensure my continued role at the facility, and I would be compensated for my time—a silver lining if ever there was one! I was thrilled to discover that I could also tackle it during the weekends. It felt like a perfect scenario: being paid to absorb invaluable knowledge about the treatment of substance abuse patients at this facility. A truly rewarding endeavor!

The ensuing weeks unfolded with a captivating rhythm as I navigated the intricacies of engaging with diverse personalities and witnessed the tumultuous journey of those striving to overcome entrenched addictions. One key realization struck me early on: substance abuse casts a wide net, ensnaring individuals from all walks of life—whether high-powered lawyers, esteemed doctors, or those living on the streets. The center where I found myself stationed was nestled in the vibrant heart of the Big Easy, a melting pot of humanity. Curiously, many inquired if I, too, was in recovery, a notion that struck me as both amusing and thought-provoking. It seemed there was an underlying assumption that my role there implied a shared struggle. The truth was, my presence was purely observational; I was collecting data and studying the manifestations of addiction. Having grappled with my own inner demons in my youth, I had forged a path of understanding and healing over the years. However, as I immersed myself in this environment, I discovered layers of complexity that far surpassed my initial expectations.

The initial weeks are particularly rigorous for these individuals. Many arrive after completing an acute detox program, where they've managed to stabilize from the severe withdrawal symptoms of their substance of choice. While some have opted for longer programs, typically lasting between 14 and 28 days, others come directly from the streets or, more recently, from local and regional jails and detention facilities. It's quite telling… Medically stable individuals are a prerequisite for commencing this rehabilitation journey. Lately, however, we've observed an increase in admissions involving patients facing significant medical challenges, which has posed quite the hurdle. As with any healthcare setting, incidents arise requiring some patients to be redirected to the hospital due to acute health crises.

Upon their entry, participants swiftly engage in the renowned "12 Step Program," a transformative initiative established in 1935 aimed at overcoming alcohol dependency, now famously recognized as Alcoholics Anonymous (AA). This journey can pose significant mental challenges for many individuals, making the initial leap particularly daunting. Herein lies the first and undeniably crucial step to embark on.

1) Acknowledge Our Limitations: We must recognize that we lack control over "alcohol, pills, etc..." and that our lives have spiraled into chaos. This step challenges many, as admitting our flaws or misjudgments is a difficult task for most of us. I've struggled with this myself. Nowadays, I can own up to my mistakes fairly well, though I recall a time in my youth when that was not the case—those days were filled with stubbornness and pride, haha.

2/3) The next two crucial steps, Finding Hope and Surrendering, hinge on faith and are deeply rooted in the divine, as yielding ourselves to God is vital for breaking free from the chains of addiction. In conversations with several patients, I've explored how those who don't share my belief in God navigate this path. They express that while some embrace faith, like I do, others find solace in the concept of karma. For many, the phrase "a power greater than themselves" can be interpreted as the Earth, science, Mother Nature, the vast universe, humanity as a whole, or even their supportive recovery community. Personally, I firmly believe that overcoming an addiction necessitates divine assistance; however, not everyone shares this view. Interestingly, some patients have confided in me that once they begin to engage with the initial steps, they find themselves opening up to the possibility of faith and developing a personal connection with Jesus. And that is precisely why we are all on this journey together!

Here are some examples of different 12 step programs that have adopted this proven treatment method:

- Narcotics Anonymous
- Cocaine Anonymous
- Crystal

- Marijuana Anonymous
- Heroin Anonymous
- Sex
- Gamblers Anonymous
- Overeaters Anonymous
- Workaholics Anonymous
- Debtors Anonymous
- Al-Anon
- Alateen
- Co-dependents Anonymous

Also, mental disorders and diseases linked to substance abuse abound! With my Healthcare/Nursing background, I've encountered some truly eye-opening situations recently, especially during my visits to patients in their homes. Witnessing the plight of individuals within the prison environment was equally enlightening. Experiencing all this firsthand in New Orleans is quite the journey. This city provides an up-close glimpse into the lives of some of the most disadvantaged and ailing individuals in the nation, grappling with the health issues spawned by the local diet and lifestyle. No place on earth boasts such a vibrant mix of festivals, famously unhealthy cuisines, Mardi Gras, bustling bars, and endless celebrations. It's a compelling concoction that brews an array of addictions and detrimental habits. One of the first people I met was a former financial advisor who, by his own admission, broke under the weight of managing a finance firm while juggling the demands of a young family. Now, he finds himself entrenched in a cycle of substance abuse that has stripped away everything he held dear. Then there was another individual, recently admitted after Mardi Gras; he was homeless, hooked on IV heroin, and had a menacing appearance. This was shaping up to be quite the experience!

Two particular personality disorders frequently coexist with substance use issues: Borderline Personality Disorder and

Antisocial Personality Disorder. Each is marked by heightened impulsivity and aggressive tendencies. Additionally, various mental health disorders may accompany substance abuse problems, including anxiety disorders, depression, ADHD, bipolar disorder, personality disorders, and schizophrenia, among others. Here's a closer look at the ten most prevalent personality disorders.

- **Antisocial personality disorder**: a pattern of disregarding or violating the rights of others. A person with antisocial personality disorder may not conform to social norms, may repeatedly lie or deceive others, or may act impulsively. Probably the most common of all.
- **Avoidant personality disorder**: a pattern of extreme shyness, feelings of inadequacy, and extreme sensitivity to criticism. People with avoidant personality disorder may be unwilling to get involved with people unless they are certain of being liked, be preoccupied with being criticized or rejected, or may view themselves as not being good enough or socially inept.
- **Borderline personality disorder:**a pattern of instability in personal relationships, intense emotions, poor self-image and impulsiveness. A person with borderline personality disorder may go to great lengths to avoid being abandoned, have repeated suicide attempts, displayed inappropriate intense anger, or have ongoing feelings of emptiness.
- **Dependent personality disorder:**a pattern of needing to be taken care of and submissive and clingy behavior. People with dependent personality disorder may have difficulty making daily decisions without reassurance from others or may feel uncomfortable or helpless when alone because of fear of inability to take care of themselves.

- **Histrionic personality disorder**: a pattern of excessive emotion and attention-seeking. People with histrionic personality disorder may be uncomfortable when they are not the center of attention, may use physical appearance to draw attention to themselves or have rapidly shifting or exaggerated emotions.
- **Narcissistic personality disorder**: a pattern of need for admiration and lack of empathy for others. A person with a narcissistic personality disorder may have a grandiose sense of self-importance, a sense of entitlement, take advantage of others or lack empathy.
- **Obsessive-compulsive personality disorder**: a pattern of preoccupation with orderliness, perfection and control. A person with obsessive-compulsive personality disorder may be overly focused on details or schedules, may work excessively, not allowing time for leisure or friends, or may be inflexible in their morality and values.
- **Paranoid personality disorder**: a pattern of being suspicious of others and seeing them as mean or spiteful. People with paranoid personality disorder often assume people will harm or deceive them and don't confide in others or become close to them. I've definitely seen this a good bit.
- **Schizoid personality disorder:**being detached from social relationships and expressing little emotion. A person with schizoid personality disorder typically does not seek close relationships, chooses to be alone and seems to not care about praise or criticism from others.
- **Schizotypal personality disorder:**a pattern of being very uncomfortable in close relationships, having distorted thinking and eccentric behavior. A person with schizotypal personality disorder may have odd beliefs or odd or peculiar behavior or speech or may have excessive social anxiety.

Here are a few, I would say, a little odder disorders I've seen in the rehab:

- Unspecified mood disorder (MDD vs Bipolar II disorder vs mood disorder due to hormone therapy), Unspecified trauma disorder, Alcohol use disorder – This individual was undergoing hormone therapy as they were transitioning from one sex to the other. I saw this a few times at the prison as well.
- Unspecified anxiety disorder, History of TBI, Opioid use disorder, Amphetamine use disorder, Benzodiazepine use disorder and Alcohol use disorder. I've interacted with the individual regularly and they are more of what you would typically see in the rehab setting these days. More of these multiple substance abuse rather than just alcohol which is like what I saw at Orleans Parish Prison.

Here are some others that can lead to substance abuse or are associated with it:

- Dissociative amnesia disorder, Bipolar I disorder, Other specified trauma or stressor related disorder. Anxiety disorder unspecified, **Opiate use disorder-on MAT** (medication-assisted treatment-typically with suboxone). ***This one is important as these individuals are getting treatment for Opioid addiction. Suboxone can help with the physical difficulties that people experience when withdrawing from an opioid. Suboxone is basically an opioid medication with the same active ingredient: buprenorphine. Only Suboxone has an additional medication called naloxone, which blocks the effects of opioid drugs. This is the main drug used in the rehab I'm at. Amphetamine use disorder, Sedative/hypnotic use disorder,

- Depersonalisation-derealisation disorder, Bipolar I disorder, Dissociative identity disorder, Other specified trauma or stressor disorder, Other specified trauma or stressor related disorder, anxiety disorder unspecified (very common), and many others.

This was an individual who arrived carrying a heavy burden: substance-induced depressive disorder, insomnia of an undefined nature, harrowing nightmares, a cocaine use disorder, an alcohol use disorder, and cannabis abuse. The sheer array of psychotropic medications required for this patient just to find even a semblance of sleep is astonishing. The takeaway here? Avoid drugs at all costs! This particular rehabilitation facility offers a lifeline to the most downtrodden, guiding them through the maze of starting treatment and assisting with the application for health insurance – often state Medicaid – which covers their care. Within the initial days of admission, they undergo a comprehensive history and physical examination alongside a psychiatric evaluation by the dedicated staff MD and psychiatrist. As I immerse myself in this environment, I discover that many of these individuals have attempted the treatment program previously, only to leave AMA - against medical advice – a choice they are free to make. As you read this, you likely have a friend or family member who has sought help for substance abuse but often stumbles on the first attempt. This program stands apart, embracing a holistic and introspective approach, paving the way for participants to atone for the harm inflicted upon themselves and those they love. For the majority, it also serves as a stepping stone toward reintegrating into the workforce.

Here are a few examples of patients who have been recently admitted to this rehab facility. Their names and identities will be excluded for privacy:

READMIT - Patient is a 47-year-old male who is self-referred to treatment and has Aetna Medicaid. Client's DOC (drug of choice) is alcohol (0/00/24 LU-Last Use date). The patient denied mental health diagnosis. The patient does have seizures with medications.

Patient is a 39-year-old male who is self-referred to treatment and has Medicaid. The patient DOC is Heroin (0/00/24 Last Use date). The patient denied medical or mental health diagnosis. Patient recently released from prison to facility for drug diversion program. The patient does go to a Methadone Clinic and is aware of the policies.

Patient is a 30-year-old male who recently discharged from… and has LHC Medicaid. Patient's drugs of choice are XTC, alcohol, and THC (0/00/24 LU date). The patient denied medical diagnosis. The patient has bipolar, schizophrenia, and anxiety with medications.

Patient is a 38-year-old female who is self-referred to treatment and has UHC Medicaid. The client DOC is Meth and Opiates (0/00/24 LU date). The patient denied medical diagnosis. Patient does have anxiety and depression with medications.

READMIT - Patient is a 43-year-old female who is self-referred to treatment and has UHC Medicaid. The patient's drug of choice is Meth (0/00/24 last use date). The patient denied medical diagnosis. Recently released from the Orleans Justice Center (New Orleans Parish Prison aka OPP). The patient does have Bipolar, Anxiety and Depression with Medications.

LATE ADMIT Patient is a 32-year-old female who is self-referred to treatment and has UHC Medicaid. Patient's drugs of choice are cocaine and alcohol (0/00/24 LU date). Recently released from a correctional facility for drug diversion program. The patient does have Hep C without medications. Patient does have Bipolar, ADD, Depression, Anxiety and Diabetes.

Ironically, three of these individuals were left-handed, and if you look at their ages, they fall right at that median age of 34 for rehab.

Based on what I have seen in this facility and talking to many of these individuals, I can safely concur that this city produces a good number of people who enter rehab multiple times. There are many temptations in the Big Easy for sure.

I have spoken with several patients who shared that before Covid, they were managing their lives as substance abusers. However, as the pandemic struck, it spiraled them deeper into addiction due to job losses, family breakdowns, and other crises. It's crucial to note that many had struggled with these demons long before Covid came calling, some tracing back to their adolescent years. Their stories often echoed the same tragic themes of loss, with many having lost everything, including their loved ones. What struck me as particularly intriguing was how my perception of their ages veered so far from reality. At 52, as I pen these words, I often catch people off guard with my age—guessing I'm younger, thanks perhaps to some decent genetics. Yet, as I interact with these patients, I find that many are far older than I would have anticipated. A few of them are in their early 40s, yet I imagined them to be in their 60s! The toll of smoking, coupled with their substance issues, has left them visibly worn and weathered. I recall a night while entering medication details into the system when a patient walked in—my initial guess was that they were between 58 and 60. To my astonishment, I discovered they were only 43! I was quite taken aback. When I turned to fellow nurses to gauge their guesses on this patient's age, they too were stunned. Thus began our informal game of estimating the ages of various individuals, each encounter leaving us more baffled than the last! Not to disparage anyone, it's just fascinating to see how the body can bear the scars of substance abuse over time. Initially, the clientele was typically in their late 20s to mid-50s, presenting minimal medical or psychiatric complications—primarily drug and alcohol concerns. But that dynamic would soon shift dramatically.

A few months in, we began to encounter patients with a wide array of medical issues, many manifesting serious psychiatric conditions. Initially, there were just a couple of diabetics when I began, but that number swiftly climbed to 8–10. By June of 2024, I administered two psychotropic injections—a procedure I had occasionally performed out in the field while attending to home health patients; yet, it marked a first for the rehab facility. For those who might not be familiar with psychotropic medications, allow me to provide some insight. While these drugs are commonly dispensed in pill form, here they were given intramuscularly, allowing for a gradual release into the bloodstream over an extended duration, typically spanning three to four weeks. The primary purpose of administering these injections was to assist those with difficulty remembering to take their daily medications or who were struggling to swallow pills or liquid forms. "Pill dysphagia" is a legitimate concern!

One particular individual stands out from the recent batch of admissions to the rehab center. They were in urgent need of their monthly injection soon after arrival and displayed a rather assertive demeanor in their demands. This patient was grappling with several substance abuse issues and also bore the weight of paranoid schizophrenia. It's not unusual to see a harmful interplay between substance abuse and schizophrenia, which complicates medication adherence; hence the necessity of the monthly injection. My interactions with similar cases date back to my days working at the jail, both before and after Hurricane Katrina. However, witnessing this in a rehab context felt distinctly different, tinged with discomfort. They wore a mask of flat affect, an unsettling emptiness in his gaze that, paradoxically, also carried an edge—a hint of menace lurking beneath the surface.

"I ain't got my shot in a minute Doc..."

"What's your name? Let me see if it's in..."

This appeared to anger the patient a little...

“They told me that shit yesterday... Damn! The last time I got my shot was a week before I went to jail and I didn't get it in there!"

Hmmm... This individual recently got out of jail... Interesting.

Now I was intrigued and a little concerned at the same time and now I had to investigate.

"Ok... When did you get out of jail, and where were you when you last got your shot if it wasn't in jail? Were you at the New Orleans Jail? Or somewhere else?"

Clearly aggravated at this point the patient blurted out "Man shit... I don't know... don't y’all know that shit?"

I had to fight the urge to snap back and did so...

"Listen... This is the first time I'm meeting you and we'll get it figured out but you gotta give me a little info first..."

After a little back and forth, I was able to let them know that the medication had been ordered and be administered tomorrow. I was also able to find out that they were in jail for getting into a fight under the I-10 near the train station in a homeless encampment area. This area is notorious for having numerous homeless people living in makeshift tents, I’ve driven past that area many times and it goes through spurts of being cleared out by the city, and then it seems to fill up again and again. Sad.

A few weeks later, in a twist of fate, I found myself making the I-10 exit by the train station one evening on my way to work at the rehab center. The road was congested, a consequence of ongoing construction, and a couple of police cars lined the street, attempting to manage the traffic. One direction veered towards the Superdome, while the other led through a glaring red light—exactly where I was headed... As I navigated the final stretch of the off-ramp, I glanced to my left beneath the overpass, and my heart sank. There, huddled together, were three or four homeless individuals, and chillingly, one of them was injecting something into his right arm! I could only assume it was heroin, though it could have easily been a concoction of anything else. Positioned merely 30 to 40 feet away, I had an unobstructed view of this stark reality. It was a jarring sight—something I'd only encountered in movies, never in the rawness of real life. As a few moments passed, it struck me that two police cars were stationed about 200 feet from the scene, idling at the red light! It was only around 4:45 PM, the sun still casting a warm glow over the city. The audacity of this seemingly homeless group, openly engaging in such acts with law enforcement so near, was astounding.

I understand this might sound unbelievable, yet if you look at this video (https://youtu.be/MHMH06bVeJw?si=RCRsUib6ojS4PUQR), it may capture a glimpse of the drug-riddled underbelly of New Orleans. As I crept away and up to the red light where the cops were directing traffic, I contemplated rolling down the window and saying something to the cop, but the light turned green, and I just eased on through and made my way to work, shaking my head. On a little side note there are a few other videos that I found fascinating to see as I was scrolling through YouTube.

Here are a couple of links to an abandoned Cold War underground bunker just a couple of miles from downtown New Orleans (https://youtu.be/NFtscLbUmZc?si=3QHQuQ9Cb4EHNVpr), (https://youtu.be/rvZsJMgxep8?si=5jA_GgQijrzUdyRu – in this one, you can see an aerial view of where the bunker is sticking out of the floodwaters of Katrina), one from an abandoned power plant on the Mississippi River near downtown (https://youtu.be/bJRweLXMkGw?si=vYjUZlG5z9eaa0Ge), and one from the well-known Charity Hospital right in the heart of downtown New Orleans (https://youtu.be/YM2iAzywUO0?si=

uQcEASe54et9XlIs). Pretty cool to watch and you just don't see things like this in bigger cities and especially after Hurricane Katrina.

I now find myself deeply entrenched in another sweltering summer in NOLA, where the rehabilitation center buzzes with activity, overflowing with individuals striving for renewal. It's intriguing—as I've mentioned before—how many left-handed patients are seeking treatment, a peculiar phenomenon that piques my curiosity. As of July 2024, the influx has only grown, with a few more “lefties” recently arriving from far and wide. This isn't mere chance... While about 10% of the global populace is left-handed, here in this place, the figure swells to nearly 30%. There's no denying it—something's afoot. Generally, we maintain an average of 65 to 70 patients, and the last tally found around 20 of them wielding their left hands. One broiling July evening, an encounter with one such left-handed patient unfolded, leading to a rather unexpected request. Just as I was preparing for the 5 PM med pass, a patient who had settled in about a month back approached me, seeking some assistance…

"Hey Doc... Can I get something for this thing that's making my right ankle itch..."

Not sure what they were talking about, I had to investigate.

"What is it?... Let me take a look..."

What I saw next threw me off a bit. When I lifted their pants leg up there was an ankle monitor with a small flashing red light looking right up at me!

"Well... ok... Where is it itching?" I can say I've never seen one of those before and I was hoping the patient didn't notice my slight surprise...

"Right here Doc... Shit is aggravating..."

Then, I went back behind the medical station to grab some gloves and some hydrocortisone cream to put on the interior region of their ankle to see if that provided some relief.

As I'm walking back, I'm just shacking my head a bit laughing to myself… I've never seen an ankle monitor up close like that. The funny thing is that the patient has been here about a month, and I had no clue they were wearing one.

"Thanks Doc… I'll be going out to a group meeting this evening… Do you think I can get my meds for the night?"

Part of this rehabilitation program entails not only the 12-step plan but also a structured progression through various phases. After an individual's initial admission and consistent weekly evaluations, they eventually earn the opportunity to attend external support meetings where they can connect with peers on the same recovery journey. I'd like to highlight the first three steps of the 12-step process, as these serve as the cornerstone for embarking on the road to recovery.

They are as follows:

- Step 1 - Acknowledge Powerlessness - This step involves acknowledging that one cannot control their addiction and that life has descended into chaos. For many, this admission proves to be one of the hardest hurdles to overcome, as it requires facing our own shortcomings and the reality that help is needed.

- Step 2 - Cultivate Hope - This step calls for the belief that a force greater than ourselves can guide us back to sanity. In my view, this conviction is essential. I've observed that individuals who struggle with belief in a higher power often encounter more challenges—those in rehab, those incarcerated, and even some who seek recovery at home appear to grapple with this concept. These individuals frequently wrestle with multiple adversities: mental health issues, medical conditions, and dependencies, often occurring simultaneously, creating a whirlwind of stress. Throughout this journey, I've gleaned invaluable insights about the human experience and its inherent imperfections, including my own. There's plenty of work ahead for me, particularly in how I can aid those I meet along the way while recognizing my own flaws in the process.

- Step 3 - Surrender - This step speaks to the commitment of entrusting our will and lives to the care of God as we understand Him. In hindsight, I wish I had embraced this idea sooner… Interestingly, the average age for first-time rehab entrants hovers around 34. I had assumed it would trend older. By their early 40s, many have experienced marriage, parenthood, divorce, and often a battle with addiction since their teenage years.

I have to say many of them return from the meeting in a good mood. I've heard them talk about this one meeting that's quite large and actually sounds fun! I'm going to try to attend one before this journey is over…

I grabbed their MAR (Medication Administration Record) to see what the meds were.

"What time will you be back from the meeting? I'll be here until about 10:30 p.m."

"About that time… the last time I came back, I couldn't get my meds… besides, I can't be out too late anyway with this damn thing on my ankle!"

We both chuckled a little bit about that, and I assured them I'd be here to give them their meds, as there were a couple in there that were best not to leave the facility.

This is where the 4th, 5th and 6th steps of the 12-step program really kick in. The meetings are where the reality of what they are trying to accomplish becomes clear. Here are those steps for those who believe that God is part of the recovery.

- Step 4 - Take Inventory - Engage in an unflinching, diligent, and sincere moral self-assessment. Those I've conversed with often assert that this is perhaps the most daunting step at the onset of this journey. The primary hurdles stem from mental obstacles and a reluctance to embrace personal accountability. This resonates deeply with our human nature; we inherently resist acknowledging our wrongdoings, and it often results in one of the gravest injustices we can inflict upon ourselves and those around us.

- Step 5 - Share Inventory – Confess to God, to our inner selves, and to another person the precise nature of our faults. This act can prove to be a formidable challenge for many, while for others, it serves as a catharsis and an awakening to the resolve required to conquer this addiction and atone for the harm caused. I've had discussions with several patients regarding this matter, and, as you might guess, some find it exceedingly tough. Personally, I've wrestled with the grip of gambling throughout my life, and the reasons evade me. There were days of exhilaration, balanced by many that were far less bright! Following my father's passing in 2014, I seemed to dive deeper into it. My mother once recounted how he would sometimes splurge his entire paycheck at the racetrack, a notion I struggled to grasp until adulthood. Yet, I can't quite pinpoint why I ventured down that path; my escapades didn't revolve around horse racing, but rather a myriad of other temptations, haha. Perhaps I inherited that tendency… Regardless, after spending time at this rehabilitation center and witnessing the struggles of these individuals firsthand, I recognize my flaws and realize the need to face myself honestly in the mirror.

- Step 6 - Become Ready – At this stage, one ought to be wholly prepared to have God eliminate all these flaws of character. Undeniably, there's a divergence between believers and non-believers in this realm. I haven't delved deeply into how others navigate this phase, but it's usually evident who possesses faith. By the time one arrives at this pivotal step, it seems they've made significant progress with the earlier two. I believe we can all embrace this step as an opportunity for collective evolution in our humanity, without a doubt.

- Step 7 - Ask God – Humbly ask Him to remove our shortcomings.

There is not much to add here.

- Step 8 – List Amends - Make a list of all the persons we have harmed and become willing to make amends to them all.

This, in my opinion, would be tough but necessary to do and from talking to some of these patients, it's right up there with Step 5 in degree of difficulty, as picking open those old wounds can trigger some challenges. However, most feel better when they have done this.

- Step 9 - Make Amends - Made direct amends to such people wherever possible, except when to do so would injure them or others.

Pretty self-explanatory there. Not all things can be forgiven, but it's good to try to make amends.

- Step 10 – Continued Inventory - Take a personal inventory, and when we are wrong, promptly admit it.

Again, a challenge from what I'm being told, but it becomes easier over time when a person is committed to quitting their addiction and recovering their life back.

- Step 11 - Pray and Meditate - Through prayer and meditation, we improve our consciousness and connect with God. We do this to understand Him, praying only for knowledge of His will for us and the power to carry it out.

The facility I'm at does this regularly with many of the individuals required to perform therapeutics as part of their day. This may range from working in the kitchen to mopping the floors to the laundry room. This helps them get back into the routine of working and contributing to the community. It's interesting to see them interact in this setting and how they react to others who may complain about the food or some other related matters.

- Step 12 – Help Others - Having a spiritual awakening as the result of these steps, we tried to carry this message to alcoholics/substance abuses, gamblers sex addicts, etc, and to practice these principles in all our affairs.

I've come across numerous individuals throughout my life who have reached this pivotal moment, but regrettably, many have stumbled along the way. However, there's a remarkable friend of mine who, at the tender age of 20, had the clarity to confront his severe struggles with alcohol and drugs. He chose the path of recovery then, and remarkably, he remains steadfast in sobriety to this day. Over the years, he has embraced the role of a "Big Brother" to countless others, guiding them with inspiring success. Now nearing 40, he continues to forge ahead, a beacon of resilience. Such strength speaks volumes in the lifelong journey of recovery—indeed, taking that first step is the most daunting challenge of all.

Chapter 6

Here We Go Once Again

As I put pen to paper, reality shifts into the realm of the surreal. Nearly two decades later, just weeks shy of the cataclysmic day, a hurricane materializes in the lower Gulf of Mexico, the date now September 7, 2024. Forecasts predict its fury to strike the Louisiana coast on a date etched in infamy: 9/11/24. Scanning the weather reports leading up to its arrival, I discovered the chilling fact: the most storms ever named in history have emerged on September 10th, with the height of the season gripping the city of New Orleans. It's almost too bizarre to fathom.

The facility reached out to me early on the morning of September 11, 2024, asking if I could cover a shift from 8:00 a.m. to 8:00 a.m., a solid 24 hours, in preparation for Hurricane Francine. Another hurricane, can you believe it? I really thought we'd avoid this season unscathed. Damn! I guess it is what it is. I managed to get my mother situated safely, yet my mind wandered to thoughts of my dad that day. This hurricane felt distinctly different from Katrina. This time, there was no dad, no wife, no dogs, no family around to distract me from worrying about anything aside from my mother, who was secure for now. I wouldn't be trapped in a prison, wondering if my dad would survive or if we'd find a way out of the chaos surrounding us. So, I packed a few essentials and arrived just before the weather began to take a turn for the worse.

If someone had told me a year ago, right as I kicked off this social experiment, that I'd find myself weathering another hurricane in a rehab facility... Well, I would've placed my bets against that, haha! It's just wild how these storms have their sights set on this region. Imagine if Florida wasn't where it is... We'd be pummeled by at least two to four hurricanes annually! New Orleans would become a ghost town! Frankly, it's edging close to that now, especially with insurance prices spiraling out of control.

Ok, I'm off my pity party now. I went to the facility, parked my car, and happened to look to my left, where I could see the New Orleans Justice Center building and the old HOD building in the distance.

I often rush through my shift at work, barely registering my surroundings as I hurry to complete the medication pass. But on this particular day, time seemed to stretch. Glancing up, I caught a glimpse of the Broad Street overpass—an almost ghostly reminder of the day my father and I had been rescued, nearly two decades ago. Waves of vivid memories crashed over me, conjuring visions of that helicopter hovering near the very spot where I now stood. I recalled the fifteen of us crammed into that chopper, each face reflecting a mix of disbelief and sheer relief at our survival. I couldn't help but wish we had smartphones back then, capable of capturing those moments. The imagery would have played like a blockbuster film, vivid and wild—a story worth telling again and again.

After a couple of minutes of flashbacks, I entered the building and clocked in on the computer.

I have not worked the daytime here before, and it is a little different, for sure. Some of these patients have outside medical appointments, and with the storm coming, some were canceled, which caused anxiety for a few of the patients.

"Damn... My doc was going to refill my script today... I need that medicine!"

Another one came in that was just admitted and a diabetic. A couple of his meds were not ordered during his transfer, these diabetics can be tricky.

"Yall got me covered on my insulin?... What about my Gabapentin? What about my…"

As I step through the door in the evenings, it seems most of the day's pressing issues are already settled. Typically, I handle medication distribution upon arrival, entering the prescriptions the doctor issued hours earlier. But today? That's a different story! Recently, we've seen an influx of patients whose medical needs are as complex as their addiction struggles. A handful of these individuals have proven exceptionally difficult. Medications seem to vanish, and patients insist they "no longer take this" or claim, "the doctor changed that..." Back when I first started, the patients' medical requirements were straightforward, but now, we face a growing number who demand intense medical attention alongside their addiction therapy.

On the morning of September 11th, 2024, I joined one other medical professional to work a shift stretching from 8:00 a.m. to 8:00 a.m. the following day, contingent on any unexpected developments after the storm subsided. Upon arrival, I roamed the facility, seeking to familiarize myself with those present, the patients who had opted for discharge in light of the storm's direct approach, and the general well-being of those remaining. They were due to return by Friday at noon, assuming there were no mega floods or fierce wind devastation to disrupt plans. Furthermore, all patients faced a mandatory drug screening upon their re-entry. The threat of leaving and slipping back into old habits loomed large, especially with the daunting reality of another hurricane bearing down, leaving chaos in its wake.

As I stepped out of the clinic, I paused to peer through the glass door into the cafeteria, where a television flickered with the familiar glow of a news broadcast—ABC, if I recalled correctly. The screen replayed the haunting footage of the first plane striking one of the towers in New York, a poignant reminder of the 23rd anniversary of 9/11. In that moment, a profound realization washed over me: I had come full circle in my life.

I was in nursing school, perhaps on my second or third day, when the unthinkable struck: we learned that a plane had crashed into the first twin tower. Just then, our instructor was maneuvering a television into our classroom. With urgency, she turned it on, and we collectively tuned into the unfolding chaos on the news. Moments later, horror escalated as the second plane collided with the second tower, and in that instant, I understood this was no accident—it was an attack. Looking back now, it feels as though this moment heralded a new age of calamities sweeping across the world…

Multiple wars in the Middle East, the massive 2004 tsunami in the Indian Ocean killing over 100,000 people, Hurricane Katrina, the Gulf of Mexico/BP Oil Spill, Covid-19, the 2023 attack on Isreal and the list go on and on… The interesting part about all of this is that it is prophesied in the Bible…

Matthew 24:6-13…

You will hear of wars and rumors of wars, but see to it that you are not alarmed. Such things must happen, but the end is still to come. Nation will rise against nation, and kingdom against kingdom.

There will be famines and earthquakes in various places. All these are the beginning of birth pains.

“Then you will be handed over to be persecuted and put to death, and you will be hated by all nations because of me (this is modern-day Israel as well). At that time, many will turn away from the faith and will betray and hate each other, and many false prophets will appear and deceive many people. Because of the increase of wickedness, the love of most will grow cold, but the one who stands firm to the end will be saved…

Luke 81:20

"When you see ISRAEL surrounded by enemies on all sides, LOOK UP, your deliverance is near."

We are in the end times, no doubt! The whole world is on fire, and this is just the beginning.

If you take a moment to truly ponder the events that followed Jesus’ crucifixion and the subsequent threads woven through history, it’s all documented in the Bible, but one must delve deeper to unearth its truths. I mention this because when I embarked on my journey at the prison back in 2003, I had just stepped into married life, finding myself distanced from the church community. My background included a Catholic high school education, but life took me to college, where my church-going days faded into memory… Fast forward to 2003; there I was, one evening in the medical clinic, my gaze landing on a Bible resting atop the desk. Curiosity piqued, I flipped it open and was drawn into the pages of Revelation. In just a couple of days, I read it twice. That initial spark ignited a fervent quest to explore the rich imagery woven throughout Revelation. Notably, the Book of Daniel parallels many of the prophecies foretold in Revelation, creating a fascinating tapestry of events. During my exploration, I encountered a remarkable man named Steve Wohlberg, who adeptly illuminates the prophecies concerning the United States within Revelation. Truly compelling insights await you. Check out this video:

(https://youtu.be/5GnZnWQKZ7w?si=ZpV9BwmPEGz1RPdf).

Apologies for the digression, but it felt essential to share. After traversing the facility and engaging with a few patients, I made my way back to the cafeteria to catch the latest weather update. The news remained grim, as Hurricane Francine barreled toward New Orleans. Ugh...I went outside after that to my car to grab my blow-up bed and bag, as I would be finding a place to set up my stuff. I agreed to work through the storm, so I came prepared. So, I thought... This is starting to feel eerily like 2005 and Hurricane Katrina, minus having my father with me. I had an idea to see if the conference room at this facility was open and set up shop in there. It wasn't that big and not occupied that often, from what I could tell. I went to the clinical administrator to see if it was okay, and permission was granted. The room was just down the hall from the medical clinic and was nice and cool for now. I went and blew up my bed just in case. If the power goes out from the storm, I wanted to be all set up.

The day crawled by with medication rounds and a smattering of minor crises to tackle, as we all sat poised for the impending storm. I had anticipated the weather to deteriorate earlier than it actually did, but when it finally turned, it was swift and severe. As twilight descended, the rain lashed down, propelled by fierce winds. I reached out to my neighbor, checking on conditions, and he replied that they had just lost power twenty minutes before my message pinged his phone. My home lies near the airport in New Orleans, a mere whisper away from the scars left by Hurricane Katrina and the battering endured from Ida. And now here comes Francine... It seems like those female hurricane names pack quite a punch, don't they?

As the storm worsened, it signaled the arrival of the 8 PM medication round. A crew accumulated at the medical clinic's entrance, each person seeking solace in the now-familiar routine. But within mere minutes, the piercing shriek of the fire alarm shattered the air —louder than any alarm I had ever experienced, catching me off guard and setting my heart racing. Oddly enough, despite the irritating sound, no one appeared particularly alarmed, myself included. The absence of smoke presented a false sense of security, leading me to suspect that something outside had somehow triggered the alert. Continuing our task uninterrupted, we doled out medications for another five minutes until the unmistakable voice of the facility's director boomed through the PA system: "This is not a drill… I repeat, this is not a drill… evacuate the building immediately!"

The wind howled ferociously outside, whipping at speeds of 80 to 100 mph, while relentless sheets of rain lashed against the building. I instructed the small crowd of people waiting anxiously in line to make their way outside. With patients and staff combined, there were easily over 60 people huddled together beneath the stormy skies. A few more might have joined us, but several patients opted to flee the facility, escaping the chaos to get out of town. Ironically, they were due to check back in that ominous Friday the 13th if they wished to continue their rehab program and would need to provide a urine sample for testing.

As we stepped out into the blackness, relief washed over us knowing that the building was elevated; a carport sheltered us beneath the second floor. Meanwhile, the Clinical Director launched into a roll call of those who were outside—a peculiar sight given the winds howling at 100 mph around us, with the fire alarm wailing like a banshee! Barely ten minutes had passed before a fire truck rumbled into the parking lot, its lights cutting through the torrential downpour. Two firefighters hopped out, nonchalant despite the rain drenching them, striding up to the facility's entrance. Inside, the administrator and another manager gathered in the lobby, standing amidst the background noise of the relentless alarm, their expressions a mix of urgency and bemusement.

We all found ourselves huddled beneath the second-floor overhang, and I must say, this was only my second experience standing out in the eye of a hurricane. The first was back in college. A few friends and I thought it would be a brilliant idea to throw a hurricane party in Lafayette, LA, during the impending chaos of Hurricane Andrew in 1992. Andrew had just wreaked havoc on Miami days before, and now it was barreling straight for Lafayette as I was gearing up for my third year at the University of Louisiana at Lafayette. In those days, we were blissfully ignorant—no cell phones, no formal evacuation plans, and FEMA was merely a name I had yet to encounter. My roommate and I boldly decided to host a hurricane gathering, inviting anyone who wanted to brave the storm with us. Armed with a two-bedroom apartment and an ample supply of beer, we embraced the thrill of the unknown. I can't recall the faces of everyone who joined us or the specifics of that wild night. The only vivid memory is of gingerly opening the front door to our second-floor apartment as the wind screamed outside, surely gusting over 100 mph. Clutching a beer in my left hand, I swung open the door just in time to see a potted plant and some kind of chair whirl past me! Instinctively, I yanked the door shut and stumbled back, the shock hitting me like a freight train - my heart racing, laughter mingling with fear, as I landed hard on my backside, completely awestruck.

Some time later, perhaps a couple of hours had slipped by, the wind began to settle, signaling the passing eye of the storm through our city. A few adventurous souls among us ventured outside, eager to experience the eerie tranquility that accompanied the storm's eye. As I draft this narrative, fragments of that moment float back to me, beer in hand, lol. I remember the sunlight piercing through the clouds, highlighting the chaotic aftermath surrounding us.

Never had I encountered such a wild scene before, where the wind and rain hammered us, only to be replaced abruptly by an uncanny stillness. It was odd. We were unsure of how long this serenity would linger, and the faces of those around me—aside from my roommate—blurred into insignificance. Yet, I recall a menacing wall of darkness looming to the south, urging us back indoors. Thus, we retreated, drinking more beers to ride out the storm's onslaught and embrace a drunken oblivion as it raged on outside... back to the rehab.

The incessant wail of the fire alarm pierced the air, reverberating through the building as we huddled together in the first-floor lobby, seeking shelter from the torrential rain that battered against the windows. The wind howled, a relentless force swirling around us. Many of us, patients included, instinctively pulled out our phones, excitement coursing through our veins as we captured this unexpected drama. Just then, the director stepped in, his voice a solid authority amid the chaos. He sternly reminded us that this was a private facility and that recording was absolutely forbidden. A chorus of frustrated groans erupted as hands grudgingly lowered phones, though a few daring souls continued to snap shots, lol. Oh well. Eventually, the fire department arrived, managing to silence the deafening alarm, but an air of uncertainty still loomed—no one had confirmed if there was truly a fire. I hadn't detected even a hint of smoke, and it appeared the firefighters were just as bewildered as we were.

We made our way back into the building just as the firetruck pulled out of the parking lot, but the alarm blared to life once more, throwing many into a frenzy! We were on the brink of restarting the medication pass when the chaos ensued, voices rising, everyone demanding the alarm be silenced. The relentless noise was driving me nuts—it felt like my ears were under siege! We hustled to speed through the med pass to avoid further annoying the patients, who were growing increasingly impatient. A few even snapped at me, as if I had flipped the switch myself. I brushed it off; I'd probably react the same way if I were in their shoes. As we began to wind down the med pass, a supervisor appeared, informing us that the fire department had clarified that the alarm had been triggered by the relentless wind and rain—no fires or electrical mayhem to report, thankfully. It made sense, but I couldn't shake the irritation that the alarm, supposedly reset, continued to blare intermittently, adding to the muddled atmosphere.

We closed the medical clinic at about 10pm as the wind, rain and fire alarm continued to go off. It was maddening! We were still available for emergencies, but the main part of our work was done for the day. 14 hours straight with a couple of breaks in between and a mini fire evacuation. I eventually made my way to the corporate board room where my sleeping arrangements and air mattress were. We still had generator power at this point which was vastly different than my last hurricane working situation. During Katrina the power went out and the generators were flooded and crashed quicky during the storm as we were plunged into darkness. Anyways, it was still comfortable in their temperature wise as I grabbed my toothbrush and toothpaste. I made my way to the clinic bathroom, but it felt more like a community bathroom. The other person with the medical team for the storm was in there when I got there so I walked over to the windows of the clinic to look outside. Of course, it was still blowing pretty hard and raining but you could tell it was just about through the city. I looked out to the right and I could barely see the right side of the Orleans Parish Prison/Orleans Justice Center through the rain.

Here I stand, nineteen years later, mere footsteps from the prison that once confined my father and me in misery. It feels almost surreal—if someone had told me I would return to this spot, I would have laughed at the absurdity. Yet here I am, the ghosts of the past whispering in my ear. After a deep breath, I make my way to the bathroom, the familiar routine grounding me in the present.

I brush my teeth and head back to my makeshift bed for the night. The power hums softly, and the Internet is a comforting constant, so I set up my laptop and log into Netflix. I need to distract myself for a while before I can brave the embrace of sleep. Good sleep has always been a fickle friend to me.

I finally drifted off to sleep with my computer humming in the background and a movie flickering on the screen. I was jolted awake by a few patients gently knocking on the conference room door, eager for their morning medications. I couldn't help but chuckle to myself—many of these patients can't survive even a single med pass without their pills. With a resigned breath, I entered the room to tackle the morning med pass. In the midst of the routine, I shot a quick text to my neighbor to check on our power situation and how our apartments had fared. The news wasn't encouraging; the floodwaters came right up to the doors of our homes, and the power was still out. Feeling the rising tide of urgency, I decided to reach out to a friend, seeing if I could find refuge at his place—no sense in heading home when it was just a short jaunt from the rehab facility. Thankfully, he answered and generously offered me his spare apartment. Life in this part of the country is a relentless struggle... Each year, we're haunted by the looming threat of a hurricane, and here we are, hit again. To be fair, it looked like it could have turned out much worse.

When the power finally came back on, I rushed home, only to discover the aftermath of chaos: my bedroom ceiling sagged ominously, the upstairs bathroom bore water stains like a sad memoir, and the laundry room downstairs looked like it had hosted a rainstorm of its own. Truly devastating… As luck would have it, only my condo and one other out of the twenty in the complex seemed to have suffered damage. I can only brace myself for yet another bout with the insurance company and the daunting search for a reliable contractor to restore my home once again.

After settling into my temporary lodgings, I found myself on call for the home health company during the weekend that followed Hurricane Francine. The early reports indicated substantial flooding across the city, though not much wind damage was noted. The patients I had to visit were scattered all over town, offering me a chance to witness the aftermath firsthand. My first delivery was to a house in the 7th Ward, not far from where I had seen that dubious drug deal transpire—the kind that makes your heart race, thinking you might be next. A flicker of caution washed over me as I approached, but I resolved that if the scene looked too unsafe, I'd just roll on by. According to her chart, I would be heading to see a 94-year-old woman who lived alone and needed her monthly psychiatric injection. I had spoken to her on the phone the night before, and although she came across as kind, you never really know what to expect.

As I approached her street the next day, the scene appeared calm, yet a few blocks before revealed disarray. It was quintessential New Orleans. Familiar with the city, I had never ventured into this particular section before. Pulling up, the general area bore the aftermath of a recent storm, with trash strewn across sidewalks, along with small branches and scattered leaves. This neighborhood showcased the signature "shotgun" houses—narrow and elongated, a relic of architectural history that piqued my curiosity. I took a moment to delve into the origin of the name, learning it stemmed from the notion that if one were to open all the doors, a bullet fired from the front could zip straight through to the back without hitting a single wall, a metaphorical "shotgun blast." The irony wasn't lost on me—New Orleans, a city entwined with tales of gunfire, was marked by homes named for weaponry. This architectural style, it said, traced its roots back to West African designs brought by Haitian slaves to the vibrant heart of the city. There it was, a nugget of knowledge gleaned amidst the chaos. I gathered that perhaps you, too, might learn a thing or two today if you hadn't heard this before. How amusing, too, that this very insight was crafted by AI lol.

Anyway, I made my way to the patient's front door and knocked on the door. After about thirty seconds or so, a male, late 30's to early 40's if I had to guess, answered the door...

"What's up man... Come on in... She's in the back..."

I thought to myself that this guy looked familiar, but I wasn't quite sure.

"Hey... Ok thanks..."

As I walked back to the patient's kitchen area, I could feel this guy looking at me. The patient was sitting at the kitchen table as I introduced myself.

"Hi ma'am... My name is Gavin and I'll be checking you out today and giving you your shot..."

She was a little lady who was fairly hunched over at the table and a little hard of hearing. She took a few seconds to respond, but eventually, she also introduced her grandson, who answered the door. He was looking at me like I should know him....

"Ms. J... did you stay for the storm, or did you evacuate?"

"Oh, I stayed... my grandson right here took good care of me..."

Before I could even respond to her, he interjected...

"You don't remember me?... Don't you work at the prison..."

I was a caught off guard a little but knew I had seen him before...

"Yeah, I thought I had seen you before but wasn't sure where. I haven't been there since February... Around Mardi Gras..."

The patient looked a little confused and said, "y'all know each other?"

"Yeah grandma... He gave me my flu shot when I was there before Christmas... I'm so glad to be out of that shithole of a place...

I figured it was something like that. I gave so many and saw so many people, but I didn't want him to think I didn't remember him.

"Yeah man, I hear ya... I worked there as long as I could but had to move on in February... I was there part-time and do this part-time as well..."

I could see the patient starting to nod off in the chair, as I simultaneously heard some lightning crack in the distance, I got her attention, checked her vital signs, and gave her the injection.

"Okay, Ms. J… Everything is looking pretty good. If you're on my schedule next week, I'll call you the day before to confirm a time…"

At about this time, her grandson walked me to the front door and thanked me for coming to check on his grandmother. It felt a little awkward as I opened the door to leave. I'm sure I was just projecting that onto myself, but I knew he knew where he had been. Some people are funny about that; I would probably feel that way, but who really knows…

"Alright my man… I'll see you around…"

It took him a second or two to respond saying "yeah alright man… see you around…"

Instinctively, I looked both ways as I walked down the few stairs leading from the house and quickly walked to my car. I wasn't taking any chances. The neighborhood and area were rough-looking, and it felt like it was about to rain. As I pulled off and made a right turn, I was nearly run off the road by a cop car that was flying down the road. He was flying with his lights on but no siren. It scared the shit out of me! From what I've been told, that usually means they are going to a crime scene where they need the element of surprise, or some major crime is actively happening. Whatever was going on, another cop car zoomed by me about ten seconds later. A few seconds later, I felt like my tire was low the way my car was riding, so I pulled over into what looked like a convenience store to check my tire. I wasn't really paying attention, but when I got out, it was as if I were in a time warp.

I couldn't believe my eyes! The gas station pump sign said $0.99! When I looked over at the front door of what I thought was an open gas convenience store, it was not. It was obviously closed and had been closed for several years. Pretty sure it was probably from Katrina with $0.99 gas, lol.

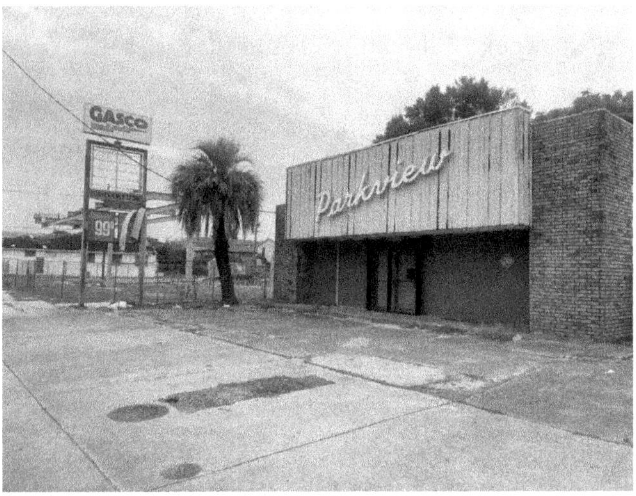

After taking in the scene for a minute, I called the rehab facility to see if I was on the work schedule for the evening. I was, so I made my way back into the city and headed to the rehab.

Wow, within a few minutes of being there, I got a call to come to the main lobby as there was a patient that literally just admitted to the facility that left to go a convenient store nearby to get a couple of things and apparently did a good bit of cocaine and was saying "I'm od'ing! I'm od'ing… (overdosing). I need to go to the ER!" Where they got it or if it was on them at the time of admit was unclear. Will be investigated, I'm sure. Well, I have never seen that before! So, as per protocol, vital signs were obtained, an incident report was filled out, an ambulance was called, and the patient was routed to the hospital for further evaluation. There were a few patients who started to hover around, but they were quickly moved by the other staff members. Once the ambulance left with the patient, it was off to do the evening med pass. The shortest admit that I've encountered so far, for sure, but I'm sure they will be back soon!

In light of this, appointments for the patients are generally arranged on a weekly basis, most often on Thursdays. Allow me to share a representative selection of patients, including the medications they are prescribed, the conditions these drugs are meant to alleviate, and their current progress. Additionally, I will provide a succinct overview of the function of each medication, along with the relevant medical terminology abbreviations. Let us begin with the first patient...

Male, early 50's-
Bipolar 1
Chronic pain secondary to MVA (Motor Vehicle Accident)
ADHD, predominantly inattentive type
Alcohol use disorder, severe
Continue Gabapentin to 600 mg TID (three times a day) as an adjunct for anxiety and alcohol cravings.

This medication is quite common in the rehab area and has many uses. Most used for pain, usually for neuropathy pain but for main types of pain in the rehab setting.

INCREASE to Duloxetine 100 mg Qam (every morning)

Duloxetine is used to treat depression and anxiety. It is also used for pain caused by nerve damage associated with diabetes (diabetic peripheral neuropathy).

Duloxetine is also used to treat fibromyalgia (muscle pain and stiffness) and chronic (long-lasting) pain that is related to muscles and bones.

Continue Atomoxetine 100 mg Qam (every morning)

Atomoxetine is used to treat attention deficit hyperactivity disorder (ADHD) to help improve attention and reduce hyperactivity and impulsiveness. As you probably already know, impulsiveness is a hallmark issue for addicts and those suffering from substance abuse issues.

Continue Mirtazapine 45 mg Qhs (at bedtime)

Mirtazapine is an antidepressant medicine. It's used to treat depression and sometimes obsessive-compulsive disorder (OCD) and anxiety. It works by increasing the amount of mood-enhancing chemicals called noradrenaline and serotonin in your brain. I didn't realize it until I started working at the rehab, as I thought it was primarily used for sleep. I've seen it a good bit over the years and just assumed it was only for sleep, but it's mainly used for depression.

Continue hydroxyzine 50 mg Qhs (at bedtime), PRN (as needed) for sleep or anxiety.

Hydroxyzine is used primarily in the rehab setting as a short-term treatment for anxiety. It's basically the same thing as Benadryl and is a very common medication for those in recovery who fight anxiety as well.

Continue magnesium oxide 400 mg Qhs (at bedtime)

***I'm highlighting this one as it was interesting to me. When I hit my mid-30s, I began to struggle with sleeping through the night. As we all know, when you have a hard time sleeping soundly, it can affect you in many ways, and it's aggravating as hell! Anyway, I asked the patient why they were on this, and they said the doctor put them on it for sleep. Magnesium helps with sleep by relaxing muscles and helping the body's natural sleep patterns. However, there isn't much research on magnesium and sleep, and the exact ways it impacts sleep are still unknown. Ironically, about a week later, my mom gave me a bottle of magnesium after she cut my hair saying she read somewhere that it helps with sleep. I was sold after that, and now I take it as well. It has improved my sleep.

Continue nicotine patch 14mg daily

Pretty self-explanatory. I'd say over 90% of rehab people smoke, and many want to try to quit smoking as well.

Continue nicotine lozenge 2mg QID (4 times a day) PRN (as needed)

Another form of smoking cessation is nicotine gum.

Here is another recent rehab admission:

Male, mid-30s.
Schizophrenia
MDD, in remission
Nightmares

Alcohol use disorder
Amphetamine use disorder
Continue Hydroxyzine 50 mg TID PRN anxiety
Continue Seroquel 150 mg Qhs for sleep

Seroquel is used to treat certain mental/mood disorders (such as schizophrenia, bipolar disorder, sudden episodes of mania or depression associated with bipolar disorder). The generic name is Quetiapine and belongs to a class of drugs known as atypical antipsychotics. It works by helping to restore the balance of certain natural substances in the brain. Unfortunately, many patients that are attempting rehab also suffer from mental disorders as well. They kind of go hand in hand.

Continue Risperdal 1 mg Qhs

Risperdal treats schizophrenia, bipolar disorder, and autism spectrum disorder. It works by balancing the levels of dopamine and serotonin in your brain, substances that help regulate mood, behaviors, and thoughts. It belongs to a group of medications called antipsychotics. I never knew that this medication was given to those on the autism spectrum. Interesting.

Paxil 10 mg q am (every morning)

Paroxetine is used to treat depression, obsessive-compulsive disorder (OCD), panic disorder, generalized anxiety disorder (GAD), social anxiety disorder (also known as social phobia), premenstrual dysphoric disorder (PMDD), and posttraumatic stress disorder (PTSD). Okay, when I saw this PMDD (premenstrual dysphoric disorder) I had to find out what it was, and I'll just say, sorry ladies, but I'm glad I'm a man!

PMDD/Premenstrual Dysphoric Disorder is a chronic mood disorder that causes severe symptoms in the week or two before menstruation:

- **Emotional symptoms**: Extreme mood shifts, irritability, anger, hopelessness, sadness, anxiety, panic attacks, feeling overwhelmed or out of control.
- **Cognitive symptoms**: Difficulty concentrating, decreased interest in normal activities.
- **Physical symptoms**: Breast tenderness, bloating, cramps, headaches, joint or muscle pain, weight gain, fatigue or low energy, food cravings or binge eating, and trouble sleeping.

PMDD is like premenstrual syndrome (PMS) but more serious. To be diagnosed with PMDD, you must have five or more symptoms, including one mood-related symptom. I wonder how many women are out there with this syndrome and how many men wish they knew what was going on with them, lol.

Continue Prazosin 1 mg Qhs for nightmares (yes, there really are meds for nightmares)

Ok, every time I look up one of these medications, it gets even more interesting… I'd only heard of Prazosin when I started working at the rehab and was under the impression this medication was only used to lessen or prevent nightmares, but check this out.

Prazosin has therapeutic uses for 5 different medical conditions. Benign Prostatic Hypertrophy (BPH), post-traumatic stress disorder (PTSD) associated nightmares, Raynaud phenomenon, pheochromocytoma (a rare adrenal gland tumor), and scorpion envenomation (getting stung by a scorpion). I looked up all 5 of these and none of them have anything to do with the other but this medication is used to treat all of them. That's crazy!! Here are the therapeutic ranges used in case you are interested. The reason I am showing these is that there was a patient at the rehab that was on 6 mg of Prazosin for nightmares and had none of these other issues. Just very strange that the same medication can have therapeutic benefits for PTSD nightmares and a scorpion sting! I guess getting stung by a scorpion might give me nightmares too! Bizarre!

The route for the administration of prazosin is oral. Doses of the medication include a 1 mg capsule, 2 mg capsule, and a 5 mg capsule.

- Hypertension treatment doses (in adults): 2 to 20 mg divided into 2 to 3 times daily doses.
- BPH treatment doses: 0.5 to 1 mg twice daily, up to 4 mg per day.
- PTSD treatment doses: Initiate at 1mg. Maintenance at 2 to 6 mg nightly. Higher doses have been used in military personnel, up to 16 mg nightly.
- Raynaud syndrome treatment doses: 1 mg three times daily.
- Scorpion envenomation treatment doses: 30 μg/kg/dose, followed by a repeat dose at 3 hours, then every 6 hours.

Anyways, I hope you find that as interesting as I do.

Continue Vivatrol shot every month, and gabapentin 100 mg qhs

This was another medication that I had never heard of until I started working at the rehab. Vivatrol is used in the treatment of alcohol dependence in patients who can abstain from alcohol in an outpatient setting prior to initiation of treatment with Vivatrol. Patients should not be actively drinking at the time of initial Vivatrol administration. I asked the patient if it was helping, and they weren't sure yet but had known a couple of people that started taking the shot and it did help with not having cravings.

My goal in sharing all of this with you is to try to paint a picture of the various things that are going on with those attempting to get better through rehabilitation.

Well, with all of that, here is a newer admit that I found interesting:

Early 40's female, who is court ordered to treatment by Plaquemines Parish Prison and does not have Medicaid. Patient's drugs of choice are heroin and meth (00/00/24 last use date). The patient has hypertension with medications. Patient also suffers from anxiety, depression, and PTSD with medications…

Well, I can say that was an interesting few days—from seeing a patient who needed a psych injection with a grandson to whom I gave a flu shot, to a new rehab admit that barely had a foot in the door and ended up at the hospital after doing a bunch of cocaine, and learning how many of the medications used today have numerous other treatment properties, to now even more hurricanes in 2024…

Within three weeks of the most recent hurricane to hit Louisiana, Francine, our region of the country, gets hit by two more, Helene/Milton, and the damage and loss of life is catastrophic. Both storms seemed to form out of nowhere and tore up several southern states. The epic flooding was like nothing seen since Katrina and had a biblical feel to it. Watching all the flooding videos and seeing the destruction was incredible. I even spoke to a buddy whose daughter just moved to Asheville, NC for college only to make her way to a fire station to avoid the flooding and eventually get evacuated back to New Orleans where she just left! Crazy!

I swear when we got past the dreadful day of 8-29 (at least six hurricanes since 2005, including Katrina, have hit the New Orleans area), which I'm now naming Hurricane Alley, I thought we were going to be good for the year. Wrong! As many times as it happens, you would think you would just get used to it, but you never really do. If you had told me almost 20 years later I'd be here writing a second book and documenting all of this, I would not have thought so...

Amid all of this, a couple of days later, I went to my damaged condo to pick up my mail, and there was a summons in the mail for jury duty. I've never received a summons for jury duty in my life. My immediate thought was to try to get out of it somehow, but soon I thought this might be interesting, especially if it were for a drug or murder charge. I mean, in the last year I've been face to face with an arson murderer of his children, kidnappers and of course many drug offenders so this might be another layer to observe in the dark side of hurricane alley!

Hmmm... I never really thought about that before, but it would be interesting if I were on a jury in a drug case or, for that matter, a murder case with some drug involvement. There is a patient at the rehab who is court-ordered to the facility, with a pending court appearance coming up soon. The only reason I know this is that a patient came in one evening a few days back and asked if they could get their morning meds for the next day, as they had to go to court for 8:00 a.m.

Given this situation, I wasn't sure if I could give the meds out, and the patient was also a diabetic, so I called the clinical administrator to check and was given the okay. The meds were given, and I was really tempted to ask what they were charged with but decided not to. I figured if they were here, then it was probably drug-related, but who knows. I'll have to try to find out.

Another intriguing facet of the rehab world is that many individuals come and go in a seemingly fleeting manner for various reasons. The rehab facility I'm currently in mandates a stay of at least 3 to 9 months, centering its efforts on the 12-step program while also working to reintegrate these patients back into the workforce and society at large. Court-ordered attendees are shackled to this place, devoid of the option to leave, but generally, anyone here has the freedom to walk away if they wish. It strikes me that many arrive eager for change or aware that they need a transformation but ultimately aren't quite prepared to make the deep commitment needed for real progress. Just the other day, I witnessed a scenario where one person was thriving in the program, only for a newcomer to arrive, and before long, both exited "AMA (against medical advice)," leaving their growth unfinished. It's disheartening to watch this unfold, as you can often see how easily some are led to abandon their path. Sadly, in my time here, two instances have been reported where someone left the facility with another person, culminating in an overdose and tragic death. I'm sure instances like these have occurred before; those are just the heartbreaking stories I've come to know.

Life is so random, especially in this rehab. Now, this is the only one I've ever worked at, so I don't have much to go on. It's now the day before Halloween 2024, and some odd stuff has happened to a few of the patients, and I'd like to share them with you.

A patient admitted about a month ago just found out a couple of days ago that his father passed away, and when I was passing his medications out the other night, he said, "The last time I was in here a few years ago, my brother passed away when I was in here as well…" Damn, what are the odds that someone's brother and father, a few years apart, would pass away when they were in the same rehab… Unreal.

Two days before Halloween, there was a patient who had worked their way through the program and gotten a job about a mile away from the rehab. It was a very foggy morning that day, and it was still dark outside. The patient was riding their bike under an overpass about two blocks from the facility when, out of nowhere, a car ran through the stop sign and hit the back tire of their bike, sending them flying onto the corner of the street and sidewalk, and the car kept going! Luckily, I guess, they only had some bumps and bruises, but the kicker was the patient didn't want to call the cops as they had a warrant out for their arrest! Wow! Luckily, they weren't killed or seriously injured, and the driver, who I still can't believe didn't stop, was lucky as hell that they didn't involve the cops due to an outstanding warrant! Crazy!

This third scenario might take the cake. The day before Halloween, I was passing medications at about 5:30 p.m., and one of the patients came in. I had heard about something they did; I had to inquire, and they confirmed it with a sheepish grin. Evidently, stealing copper is lucrative and common in New Orleans. After hearing these two stories, I had to investigate further!

There are a ton of various copper crimes, but here's one that was crazy to me. This is from March of 2024 - (https://www.wdsu.com/article/copper-thefts-i-10-nola-neworleans-city-interstate-lights/60142810). When the copper is stolen, the next thing you know, there are miles and miles of lights out—and millions of dollars spent to repair and replace. The previous summer, an investigation revealed numerous images of stolen poles, cut wiring and ripped-off copper on interstate lights. They are stealing entire interstate poles! Wild! Now back to these 2 stories here.

This patient, on this day, came to the medical unit to get their medication. I had to inquire... With a bit of a smile and a tone of voice just above a whisper, I said...

"Hey what's up... I heard you are a YouTube hit now..."

With a little smile but a remorseful look...

"Yeah doc (I get called doc a lot, lol)... Not sure what to think about that... I mean... I'm here trying to get my life straight and get clean, and now this is out there, but it is kind of funny, I guess..."

This patient has been here for a couple of months and was very quiet in the beginning but is coming out of their shell some. Ironically, they had an ankle monitor on admission, and now I know why. I could sense that they were carrying plenty of remorse, and I wanted to make sure they knew that.

"I hear ya... You are on the right path... I've seen an improvement in your overall demeanor since you got here..."

There were a few seconds of silence, and then they laughed a little.

"Yeah, it is pretty funny, I guess... I could be sitting in jail..."

I was wondering about that, and I felt like they were giving me an opening to ask...

"Yeah... I was wondering about that... Did you get a lot of time for that?"

"Actually, no... Mainly restitution... about $40,000..."

Wow... my initial thought is, how is this homeless patient going to pay back that kind of money? As I looked into it, when someone commits a crime like this, and restitution is involved, the perpetrator has to pay the restitution to the city or the state, or both, depending on who was the arresting party. It is 2024, I thought... Maybe they will become a YouTube hit and make a bunch of money!

Anyway, as this patient was finishing up their copper theft story, another patient came in, heard us, and proceeded to tell me their copper theft story! Damn, lol. Just before that, the patient blurted out, "Yeah, that's my dog right there out in the streets... I was out there doing the same damn thing..."

A little blown away by this 30-second, three-way interaction between the three of us, I had to compose my thoughts for a few seconds. I've seen both individuals at various times during my time here and can't remember a time when they were both in here at the same time, and now they are in here at the same time telling me that before coming in here, they were both committing the same type of crimes. I couldn't make this up if I tried! As the first patient went to walk out, he did a little fist bump, and I handed the medication to the second patient. He then proceeded to tell me about his copper crimes...

"Yeah G (that's what they called me)... I got caught on the 20th floor at Charity Hospital..."

I have to say, I misinterpreted what he said, thinking they were a patient admitted to the hospital when they finally caught up with them, feeling a little stupid for a second. Lol.

"Charity hospital? Been closed since Katrina... Don't you mean University hospital?"

"No G... I was living inside the hospital and was pulling copper out of the wall on the 20th floor, and they got me..."

Laughing, I said "I'm thinking for a second that you were in a hospital bed when they finally caught you and you're telling me you were living in an abandoned hospital, snatching copper when they caught you..."

It gets better. They then proceeded to tell me more.

"Mr. G... For about 4 years straight, I would go to the same... hospital..." and pull out about a $100 worth of copper a day and go sell it and never got caught..."

Full disclosure... This was a different abandoned hospital in New Orleans than the one they were talking about. I don't really feel the need to mention which one it was. Post-Hurricane Katrina, there are numerous buildings and multiple hospitals that were abandoned. I remember coming back into the city about six weeks later and going back to work at the prison. It was mainly in a cleanup capacity to begin with, but seeing all the devastation up close was remarkable. It truly looked like a nuclear bomb went off near the jail. I remember having to share a car with my then-wife and waiting for her to pick me up one evening on Tulane Ave. near the courthouse. Everything was covered in a whitish film, and you could see different water lines on the buildings, with cars still flipped over and debris everywhere from the flooding. I remember just sitting on the curb, looking around in amazement at all the destruction. I can still visualize it like it was yesterday.

After this patient told me about his copper escapades, I started doing a little math. $100 a day, tax free, for a homeless person with no bills is damn good! To do that for about 4 years and not get caught is remarkable! Over $100,000 no taxes… Even more, it's hard to believe there is that much copper in one building, let alone all buildings everywhere. There is another layer to this as well.

I was telling an old friend, whom I've known since I was 12 years old, about these two and their stolen copper escapades. We play golf together and a couple of tournaments every year. He begins to laugh when I start to tell him about this. He is in the power/electric business and proceeds to tell me about a couple of different jobs he was on in the last year or so, where he met workers involved with stolen copper. What the hell is going on!

He said there were a few groups of guys that were on this big job, and a couple of them decided to steal some of the copper and sell it. Well, my patient back at the rehab was taking smaller amounts and selling them, getting away with it for years, but these fellas went for the jugular. Just like most things, the smaller, the easier it is to get away with, but bringing thousands of dollars' worth will certainly raise a red flag. They even got away with it a couple of times, but one of them got greedy. He showed up with well over $20,000 worth of copper to sell, and they questioned where he got it from. He said he was a contractor and had more than he needed. They basically knew he was lying, and the crazy part is that you must use your driver's license and info on bigger amounts like that, and wouldn't you know it, he was caught and arrested. Interestingly, he too only had to pay restitution and not even the full amount. There was close to $50,000 in copper and only low 20's in restitution. I guess copper thieves come in all shapes and sizes!

Back to the last patient at the rehab. During the last 20 years or so, they told me they went from being in the Navy to working security, to working in a strip club, to being homeless, living in abandoned buildings stealing copper. Now in rehab, they are getting clean so they can one day see their daughter again. You can tell the patient served in the military as they were very respectful when addressing me and others, from what I could tell. Like many of these patients, at some point, they got deep into drugs and alcohol and spiraled out of control to the point of being homeless. Now, this case appeared to be one of the more severe cases, as this individual was living in abandoned buildings, stealing copper to get drugs and survive. I could tell that this was a good person deep down but just had some severe demons to overcome.

“Yeah Mr. G… I’m getting better and am on the right track… I hope to see my daughter and brother soon one day…”

I truly felt that this patient was genuine in what they were saying and feeling.

“Yes, I can certainly see that you are getting better and feeling better about yourself… How old is your daughter?”

With a remorseful chuckle, the patient said “I’m not exactly sure, but she's about 12 years old… I know it's pretty sad G… but my goal is to get my life together and get to know her…"

Wow… I'm guessing that is not uncommon, but it's still a little hard to hear. I sure hope they make it through the program…

Not a few days later, as I'm writing this book, there was a news story (https://youtu.be/j38K-4jMRU0?si=mZXS4ncdHh-etaWC) about the very facility we were talking about, Lindy Boggs (Mercy Hospital) and the future plans for it. The facility has been closed since Hurricane Katrina where 19 people died in the agonizing days after the storm. Currently, a local architecture firm owns the dilapidated building. The most recent plans for the facility was to convert it to a senior living complex with multiple facilities within the structure but those plans were scrapped as of November 2024. Now, the architecture firm is currently paying between $30-40,000 a month to maintain the building, which is insane to me. They went on to say it would cost about $3,500,000 to demolish it, but it's considered a historical land site so that probably won't happen any time soon, if at all.

Here is another video (https://youtu.be/j38K-4jMRU0?si= mZXS4ncdHh-etaWC) post Katrina that shows the devastation and confirms the vagrants,homeless, and drug addicts living there for years. It also confirms the patients' stories about stealing copper out of there for years to feed their drug addiction. Believe it or not, there are numerous buildings all over New Orleans that are in the same position. I can't imagine there is another city in the world with as many deserted historical buildings as New Orleans.

A few weeks later, we're into mid to late November, and there is still some tropical storm activity popping up in the lower Caribbean and making noise in the Gulf of Mexico. I'm so ready for some cool weather!

I decided to reach out to the Orleans Parish Prison to see if they had any availability. After seeing a few patients come here as part of a drug diversion program, my curiosity peaked again. I needed to get inside and see if things had gotten better or worse since this time last year. There was a patient who was in rehab as part of a diversion program, was of course, left-handed, and had an ankle monitor on their right ankle. They also had a money-type symbol tattooed on their left hand between the thumb and index finger. This seemed like a perfect opportunity to let them know what I had discovered, and their response was a bit shocking.

"Yes sir! I would estimate that approximately 75% of the inmates who were on the same tier as me were left-handed… when you're in jail you have a lot of idle time, and although I didn't notice it at first… it didn't take long for me to notice it after…"

Not that I didn't believe them, but I'd be trying to get a shift or two to see for myself.

The dynamic has changed some, for sure, and after my discovery of left-handedness and the criminal element to it, I wanted to see how many of the criminals were left-handed. I didn't tell anyone that I was thinking about going back undercover to continue my investigations until now.

Chapter 7

The End Game...

It had been several months since my last shift at the prison, and I hesitated, unsure if I could integrate myself back into the chaos of schedules and routines. As Thanksgiving approached, the air thick with nostalgia and loss, the city had been rattled by a series of heartbreaking events. The most devastating was a mass shooting in New Orleans. I had been on call that fateful weekend, having just finished attending to a patient nearly a mile from the scene of the carnage. It was around 4 p.m. on November 17th, 2024, a time when the city buzzed with excitement yet was equally shadowed by its gritty reality. Having lived here all my life, aside from my college years, I had long been aware of the vibrant "2nd line" parades and parties that decorated the streets, though I had never partaken in one myself. On that day, my schedule included only two patients, but I remained on standby for any emergencies that might arise. Shockingly, this marked the second mass shooting in the city during a mere year—the first occurring in April at a club in the Warehouse District, where one person lost their life and eleven others were injured. The tragedy on November 17th claimed two lives and left thirteen wounded. To compound the city's grief, just days later, a 15-year-old was arrested for shooting another teenager in New Orleans East. In this city, no place is immune to crime; it feels like all neighborhoods are intertwined in a web of violence and despair. Here I was, caring for patients in affluent homes, yet just blocks away lurked the haunting specter of crime. Preparations buzzed around the city in anticipation of the Super Bowl in February 2025, yet somehow, the city seemed unable to escape the clutches of its darker side.

A few days after this, there was an execution-style shooting in the heart of the French Quarter, with one dead and several hit by gunfire. Here is the link to the story. A famous New Orleans restaurant took on unintended gunfire as well. https://www.fox8live.com/2024/11/21/nopd-arrests-one-seeks-two-others-targeted-french-quarter-shooting-that-left-1-dead-3-injured/.

I was able to get on the schedule for Wednesday evening before Thanksgiving. This is a busy day in the city of New Orleans, as many restaurants and facilities now serve Thanksgiving meals, and given what just happened, it could be an interesting night at the jail. I'm also off on Wednesdays from the rehab facility, so this will work out just right. My goal with this shift is to see how many left-handers I encounter and if I end up in front of any of these recent shooting suspects. It would be a bonus to find out if any of them are left-handed.

As I approached the prison, a wave of disbelief washed over me; I never imagined I would find myself stepping foot in this place again. Over the past year, I've delved deeply into the intricacies of New Orleans—venturing into patients' homes, navigating the cramped quarters of their apartments, and exploring the stark reality of addiction and despair in the prison and rehabs alike, as many seek to rise from their lowest points. This time, however, my purpose for returning to the infamous Orleans Parish Prison is twofold: I aim to uncover whether the statistics reveal a greater prevalence of left-handed individuals among inmates compared to those in rehabilitation. I also seek an audience with one of the suspects linked to the latest surge of violence in the city, hoping to glean insight from their perspective amid the turmoil.

Just for a little perspective, here are a few of the most recent admits to the rehab where I worked the next day:

- Patient is a male who is referred to treatment by a detention center in central Louisiana. The patient was involved in a high-speed chase and was pulled over and found in possession of drugs among other charges. The patient is an IV fentanyl drug user (00/00/24 last use date). Patient denied and medical diagnosis. The patient does have depression and insomnia for which he takes medications.
- Patient is a 27-year-old female who is court ordered to treatment and has Aetna Medicaid. The patient denied any medical diagnosis. The patient does have ADHD and Bipolar with medications. Client DOC (drug of choice) are meth, heroin, and Xanax (00/00/24 last use date).
- Patient is a 65-year-old male who is referred to treatment by another facility and has Healthy Blue Medicaid and Medicare. The patient's drug of choice is cocaine (00/00/24 LU date). patient denied any medical diagnosis. Patient is bipolar and is currently homeless.

As you can see, the ages are wide and one questionable or bad decision can land anyone in jail. There seems to be more of an effort to rehabilitate some of these individuals rather than keeping them in jail. It does appear that most must hit rock bottom before they get help or are court-ordered to do so…

The day before I was to work at the prison, I was working at the rehab and there was a flyer on the community wall that caught my attention. There was a local AA (Alcohol Anonymous) group that was sponsoring a meeting on 11-30-24 called "Campfire Sessions" where the speakers were talking specifically about Steps 4 and 5 of the 12 Step "AA" process. At this meeting they were going to be doing "resentment burning", S'mores, and showing the movie "The night before Christmas." I must admit I don't know a lot about the 12 steps and have been learning about them during these last few months. Here are steps 4 and 5…

Step 4 of the 12-step program encourages one to make a "searching and fearless moral inventory" of themselves. This involves identifying our problems and getting a clear picture of how our behavior has affected ourselves and others around us to proceed to recovery.

I'm not, nor have I ever been in recovery but I can see how this would be challenging for most to do. This goes back to human nature as it's difficult for most to admit they were wrong. I observe it a good bit in the rehab and life for that matter and when I was younger that was a challenge. As I've gotten older that is easier to do. For someone who must do this to rehabilitate themselves and permanently change their lives it must be tough.

Step 5 of Alcoholics Anonymous, commonly known as the "Confession" step, encourages members to acknowledge their struggles and whatever harm they caused to themselves and others in pursuit of alcohol. Step 5 of AA reads that one, "admitted to God, to oneself, and to another human being the exact nature of our wrongs."

This one really grabbed my attention and made me laugh at the same time. How many times have you tried to bargain with God when you really want something or are hoping something bad doesn't happen? I'm guilty of this a lot, lol. I often feel like God knows what I'm about to ask for or borderline beg for and often doesn't go my way. I can only assume He's waiting for me to give an honest or "truly confess" the error of my ways. For an addict to truly do these 2 steps it has to be difficult but necessary.

I think I'm going to go to this to observe the various human interactions and to see how the two speakers present these steps. This should be interesting. I'll let you know what I find out. Now, back to the prison…

As I mentioned before, it has been quite a few months since I was there; there is now a new healthcare management company running the medical department. It's all quite different from when I was first here in 2003. It was a chilly evening in late November 2024 when I parked my car and made my way to the security door. Back in the day, they would buzz you in, and now you have a scan badge that gets you to the elevator to go through the body scanner at the main entrance. On this day, I will be in IPC (Intake Processing Center) for a couple of hours then up to the 2nd floor medical unit to most likely do a medication pass or the Detox patients. More than likely, it may be a combination of both.

I came in right before they shut down the IPC for about an hour to do shift change. Everything is from 7 a.m. to 7:30 p.m. to give everyone a chance to switch over and give reportthe next shift coming on. Even the cops don't bring in new arrests between 6:00 pm and 7:00 pm. If they do it's rare and the new inmate has to sit in a holding cell until the next shift is ready to go. I knew I probably wasn't going to be in IPC too long, as after being there about 20 minutes, there was a call down from the 2nd floor clinic looking to see if anyone wanted to stay and help out. There was a callout for the night shift. Some things never change.

As I was sitting there, a backup call was announced over the IPC system to one of the holding cells. One of the other nurses grabbed the Emergency Bag and we all went with a few backup deputies to the area to see what was going on. To my surprise, I immediately recognized the individual that was lying on his side, appearing to be passed out or not responding to verbal stimuli. He was recently been discharged from the rehab I work at, and he was a problem there as well. He was only at the rehab for a couple of weeks, I believe, and he supposedly had a doctor's appointment one day and instead went out drinking instead… He came back to the rehab hammered! The protocol for all patients in the rehab is that everyone gets a UDS (drug screen) upon return to the facility. If they are suspected of being intoxicated or smelling of alcohol, they get a mouth swab that will instantly reveal if they have been drinking or not. This guy was obviously drunk and slurring his words, but a swab and tox screen still had to be administered. This was only the second time I had seen this happen since I had been there, but I'm only there in a part-time capacity, so I'm assuming it happens from time to time.

The funny thing about this guy was he was kind of rude to the facility assistant doing the drug and alcohol screening saying "I haven't been drinking... Y'all can check me... whatever..."

He was so drunk, and he looked and smelled like he had just left Bourbon Street lol. The good thing about this facility/rehab program is that if/when a patient slips up, they do give them a second chance, but they must admit they drank or took something. I did see someone else in a similar situation to this be indignant and deny that they had done anything wrong, and they were discharged.

There won't be any discharging from jail… As he lay there, he began to lift himself up some appearing as if he had no clue where he was. There were about 12-15 people standing around him when you included the nursing staff, deputies and the couple of new inmates all looking at his individual try to get himself up. There were a couple of chuckles in the background after it appeared that this fella was ok. I kind of stepped back as I really didn't want this guy to recognize me. I really didn't think he would, as I only interacted with him a couple of times, but I wanted to keep a low profile for obvious reasons…

We were able to get this individual up and over to the medical clinic for further evaluation. He may have had a seizure, ingested some drugs before he got arrested… Who knows…

Vital signs were obtained along with some of his medical history. Come to find out, he had a history of seizures, and he hadn't had his medication in a "few weeks…" The nurse practitioner on call was notified, and a loading dose of his seizure medications was ordered, with a follow-up appointment with the MD in clinic the following day.

The rest of the shift, I was primarily up in the 2nd floor clinic doing the detox protocol, and out of the 23 people for that rotation, 9 were left-handed, with 2 of the 6 females being left-handed as well. That's about the ratio I've seen in the rehab as well. A couple of the individuals I had to ask if they were left-handed, but the rest I could tell by the way they got their meds. I did help with one of the medication passes. Based on the way they would take their meds or get their insulin I could tell if they were right or left-handed. Sometimes I would say, "Southpaw..." or "Lefty, I see..."

Sure enough, there is a higher ratio of left-handed people in the incarcerated environment. The world population of left-handed people is about 10%. In the incarcerated and rehab world, it's at least double that. I'd love to see an in-depth study on this in the future.

I was off the next day and that weekend. It was Thanksgiving, and when I went back to work at the rehab that following Monday, I heard about a wild event that went down on Saturday.

A fight between a practically deaf guy and another guy in rehab with an ankle monitor looking at significant prison time. Evidently, the ankle monitor guy had been picking on the deaf guy for the last couple of weeks, and he finally snapped. All of this was caught on camera. When I eventually watched it, it was kind of funny at first, and I'll do my best to describe it.

These two were just finishing breakfast, and the deaf guy had some sort of wire and got in front of the other guy. I couldn't hear it on the video, but the deaf guy was telling the other guy, "I'm gonna kill you... I'm gonna kill you..." as he was slowly wrapping the cord/wire around his hands. The other guy put his hands up, ready to throw some punches, and this didn't even faze the deaf guy as he continued to slowly wrap and tighten the grip on the cord. It became clear to me that he may have done this before! He was way too calm in the way he was doing that. A few seconds later, he lunged at the other guy as he started throwing punches. Some of the others saw this and tried to break it up as both fell against the wall, with the deaf guy continuing to try and wrap the cord around his neck. It was chaotic for a minute or so until they were about to separate them. If I were the guy with the ankle monitor, I would have walked away! This could damage his chances of reducing whatever time he is looking at I would think! Then again, if someone was trying to choke me to death I'd be fighting back as well! By the time I came back to work on that Monday both had been discharged from the facility with the deaf guy escorted out of the facility by the NOPD (New Orleans Police Department).

On that Monday evening, there was an interesting admission. She was a 63-year-old lady who was seeking treatment for a crack addiction. Clearly, this is something you don't see every day. Evidently, she was living in some sort of crack house and was able to get out of there and make her way into the facility. Pretty wild... Hopefully, she can get the treatment she needs and work the program...

On that note, I found this diagram and information below on the chemically dependent family/person. It's pretty interesting. I'm sure we all know someone or multiple people and families that fall into these categories. I left some space for those of you who might want to take notes or refer to this information. You never know…

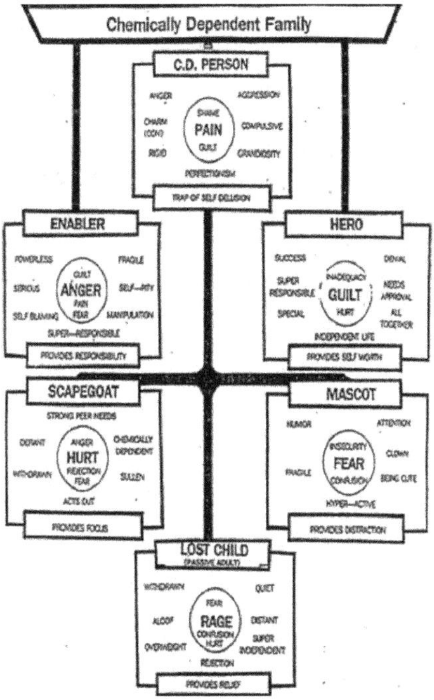

PATTERNS AND CHARACTERISTICS OF CODEPENDENCY

DENIAL PATTERNS

CODEPENDENTS OFTEN…

Have difficulty identifying what they are feeling.

Minimize, alter, or deny how they truly feel.

Perceive themselves as completely unselfish and dedicated to the wellbeing of others.

Lack empathy for the feelings and needs of others.

Label others with their negative traits.

Think they can take care of themselves without any help from others.

Mask pain in various ways such as anger, humor, or isolation.

Express negativity or aggression in indirect and passive ways

Do not recognize the unavailability of those people to whom they are attracted.

LOW SELF-ESTEEM PATTERNS

CODEPENDENTS OFTEN...

Have difficulty making decisions.

Judge what they think, say, or do harshly, as never good enough.

Are embarrassed to receive recognition, praise, or gifts.

Value others' approval of their thinking, feelings, and behavior over their own.

Do not perceive themselves as lovable or worthwhile people.

Seek recognition and praise to overcome feeling less than.

Have difficulty admitting a mistake.

Need to appear to be right in the eyes of others and may even lie to look good.

Are unable to identify or ask for what they need and want.

Perceive themselves as superior to others.

Look to others to provide their sense of safety.

Have difficulty getting started, meeting deadlines, and completing projects.

Have trouble setting healthy priorities and boundaries.

COMPLIANCE PATTERNS

CODEPENDENTS OFTEN...

Are extremely loyal, remaining in harmful situations too long.

Compromise their own values and integrity to avoid rejection or anger.

Put aside their own interests to do what others want.

Are hypervigilant regarding the feelings of others and take on those feelings.

Are afraid to express their beliefs, opinions, and feelings when they differ from those of others.

Accept sexual attention when they want love.

Make decisions without regard for the consequences.

Give up their truth to gain the approval of others or to avoid change.

CONTROL PATTERNS

CODEPENDENTS OFTEN...

Believe people are incapable of taking care of themselves.

Attempt to convince others what to think, do, or feel.

Freely offer advice and direction without being asked.

Become resentful when others decline their help or reject their advice.

Lavish gifts and favors on those they want to influence.

Use sexual attention to gain approval and acceptance.

Must feel needed to have a relationship with others.

Demand that their needs be met by others.

Use charm and charisma to convince others of their capacity to be caring and compassionate.

Use blame and shame to exploit others emotionally.

Refuse to cooperate, compromise, or negotiate.

Adopt an attitude of indifference, helplessness, authority, or rage to manipulate outcomes.

Use recovery jargon to control the behavior of others.

Pretend to agree with others to get what they want.

AVOIDANCE PATTERNS

CODEPENDENTS

Act in ways that invite others to reject, shame, or express anger toward them.

Judge harshly what others think, say, or do.

Avoid emotional, physical, or sexual intimacy to maintain distance.

Allow addictions to people, places, and things to distract them from achieving intimacy in relationships.

Use indirect or evasive communication to avoid conflict or confrontation.

Diminish their capacity to have healthy relationships by declining to use the tools of recovery.

Suppress their feelings or needs to avoid feeling vulnerable.

Pull people toward them, but when others get close, push them away.

Refuse to give up their self-will to avoid surrendering to a power greater than themselves.

Believe displays of emotion are a sign of weakness.

Withhold expressions of appreciation.

Interacting with a diverse array of patients in their own homes, within rehabilitation settings, and even in the stark confines of jails has been undeniably fascinating. From the opulent mansions to the grim jail cells, the healthcare landscape reveals a profound truth: it does not discriminate. Particularly with older individuals, the irony stands evident as they are all insured by the same entities, yet their financial circumstances and socio-economic backgrounds couldn't be more different. New Orleans, with its distinctive character, highlights this diversity vividly—something I've pointed out before. As I pen this during the holiday season, a somber cloud looms over me; a tragic event unfolded. One of my patients, who had successfully completed the 12-step program, found employment and seemed to flourish, sadly took their own life. The facility I am part of is dedicated to the long-term journey of recovery, aiding those who transition from the throes of addiction to embracing the 12-step process, securing jobs, and finding stable housing, all in a bid to reintegrate back into society as smoothly as possible.

From what I've noticed, a troubling pattern emerges among these individuals. They often become too cozy within the program's protective walls, and as the time to reintegrate into the daunting "real world" approaches, anxiety creeps in. I can see it swirling in their eyes and feel it in their fidgeting hands. Lately, a handful of them have faced the impending deadline of their stay, and unfortunately, trouble finds them. Just the other night, one patient, who had always been among the kindest and most courteous I've met, suddenly erupted, declaring that they felt homicidal and issuing threats toward another resident. This swift descent into chaos led to an emergency transfer for a psychiatric evaluation. Their struggle stands as a stark reminder that even the gentlest spirits can unearth turmoil when the safety of this environment is stripped away.

Three meals each day, a cozy room, the comfort of not worrying about bills, and the chance for social interaction, should one choose it—such a life can appear enticing. Yet, this is the same person who, not long ago, attempted to strangle another patient. The daunting reality of seeking employment, paying rent, and managing everyday expenses can be unbearable for many. Some of these individuals have transitioned from prison to rehabilitation, embarking on a challenging journey toward sobriety. The prospect of working, mending relationships with those they've harmed, and adjusting to a new way of living can weigh heavily on their shoulders.

It is now December 2024, and a deeply unsettling saga has reached its abrupt conclusion. I found myself confronted by an embodiment of pure evil, a figure whose depths of depravity are nearly indescribable. Recently, an eye-opening one-hour documentary unveiled the horrifying atrocities committed by this priest and others, revealing a systematic cover-up by the Catholic Church in the greater New Orleans area that spanned decades. At last, this individual—and I suspect several others—may soon face the consequences they deserve.

https://youtu.be/jmhhWsqRAbU?si=pf9ZJq0sAbWnXjOE

Lawrence Hecker unexpectedly entered a guilty plea on December 3, 2024, just as the trial was about to commence. This outcome took everyone by surprise, leaving the District Attorney visibly disheartened that the case would not be heard in court. The evidence assembled against Hecker was not only overwhelming but also profoundly troubling, indicating that the defendant was unwilling to endure the courtroom proceedings. Now, at the age of 93, Hecker has recently been moved to a senior living facility where he remains under tight security due to his deteriorating health. He faces an impending life sentence, potentially at the infamous Angola State Penitentiary. This case has been postponed repeatedly, plagued by various issues, most notably the defendant's diagnosed dementia. While it's likely he will stay in his current location, he is now formally convicted of the numerous rapes he perpetrated.

When I crossed paths with him at the Orleans Parish Prison, he was confined to the lockdown unit, appearing frail and withered. At the time, I was merely dispensing medications, unaware of the stormy past that had brought him there. It wasn't until later that evening, when another nurse whispered the details, that I grasped the gravity of his situation. It struck me as odd when he approached the cell door, and the deputy swung open the small slot. My first thoughts whirled—this elderly figure in a maximum-security unit looked so out of place, a striking contrast to the image of a typical inmate. He accepted his medication quietly, and as the secure hatch clinked shut, he shuffled back to his bunk, a haunting image of fragility in a world so harsh.

Even at that moment, the true depth of his actions remained an unsettling mystery, as did the vast reach of the cover-up surrounding them. To contemplate that this could occur, that it was even a conceivable reality, is utterly astonishing! I recall a segment in the documentary (https://youtu.be/jmhhWsqRAbU?si=HzK9GiKZc_uipuGD) featuring a recorded deposition, where he faced intense questioning under oath, invoking his right to remain silent over a hundred times. The inquiries were damning, and you could sense his inner turmoil; he yearned to respond but was evidently instructed by his legal team to stay quiet. It was in that instant that the past fifteen months crystallized for me. When I first embarked on this journey, I envisioned beginning in the prison and visiting patients in their homes. Never did I imagine I would encounter a man who had ignited a fire while his children slept, leading to their tragic deaths, nor meet one of history's most notorious pedophiles. The sheer absurdity of it all was overwhelming. My intention was to record the disparities between my initial days at the prison in 2003 and the present, the alarming rise of drug-related offenders within the system, and the (often painful) overlap that existed between the two. The rehabilitation aspect materialized after I commenced my work and seemed to fit seamlessly into this narrative.

Encountering both the affluent patients and those from the impoverished sectors of New Orleans on the same day has been nothing short of eye-opening. Transitioning from the door answered by an upscale nanny to keeping my head on a swivel to avoid potential carjackings has shifted my perspective dramatically. Along the way, I've mingled with everyone from homeless meth users to once-successful businesspeople now trapped in the grips of addiction. It's a complex tapestry of lives, and in this journey, I've stumbled upon the curious fact that left-handed individuals face higher rates of substance abuse issues for various reasons. It's astonishing to learn that among the general population, about 10% are left-handed; yet within the confines of rehab and prison, that figure swells to nearly double or even triple. The statistics are unnervingly consistent across these settings, prompting contemplation about the connection between left-handedness and the brain's functioning, suggesting a greater susceptibility not only to addiction but also to criminal behaviors.

I was driving to the rehab in the evening in mid-December, listening to the radio, and the head of the New Orleans Metro Crime Commission was being interviewed. The topic of conversation was quite interesting. They were talking about some crime statistics (check out this website - https://metrocrime.org/ -) that the Orleans Parish Prison was dealing with. The jail is beyond capacity, filled with violent felons. The Metro Crime Commission's website shows the different types of violent crimes, the current trends of the types of crimes being committed, and the number of inmates who committed the crimes from 2019 to December 2024. The four main crimes being tracked are homicides, shootings, armed robberies, and carjackings. The Metro Crime Commission tracked these crimes from 2019 to December 15th 2024 (see website - https://metrocrime.org/) and they peaked in 2021 and 2022, in the height of the post Covid era and Biden presidency when there was the perception of "defund the police" as a possible way of the future. Currently, there are still numerous cases awaiting trial that are backlogged due to the Covid pandemic, which is creating a huge problem. At the same time, there is a new approach to making the court system more transparent; check this out: (https://sse.tulane.edu/tulane-researchers-partner-court-watch-nola-boost-criminal-justice-transparency) that is AI based and could revolutionize the transparency of court systems everywhere. It is well documented that New Orleans has a high rate of incarceration, and the crimes are getting more violent.

During the height of Hurricane Katrina, the Orleans Parish Prison system found itself overflowing, with inmate numbers soaring to between 6,000 and 7,000. Today, that figure has diminished significantly. While a new building is in the works, it will be quite some time before it can be put to use, leaving the current issues unresolved. Perhaps it's mere coincidence, but I sense a deeper connection here. Having observed many of these individuals firsthand, I can attest to a palpable disdain for law enforcement and their legitimate authority. The pervasive disrespect within the prison system is striking; while this doesn't encompass every incarcerated individual, the situation has deteriorated since 2003. What was once an anomaly has morphed into the prevailing attitude. In recent months, I've witnessed more violent encounters, hostile actions toward medical personnel, and overall inmate aggression toward deputies combined than I had seen over the years prior. The deputies today are younger, lacking experience, and are thrust into an environment marked by audacity and aggression, all while operating under looser regulations than before. It's a troubling reality that simply doesn't add up.

With the overcrowding of the Orleans Parish Prison system, I've seen an uptick in the number of drug offenders coming to the rehab that I'm working at as part of a court-ordered measure. They are coming in regionally from various correctional facilities. Needless to say, some of the individuals are not really there to get better. They are there to avoid longer prison sentences, and if I was in that situation, I can't say I wouldn't do the same thing.

Something that has happened recently has caught my attention. There has been a bit of a younger criminal element being admitted to the rehab. There have been a few 19-to-24-year-olds with recent drug arrests who have made their way to the rehab via the court system. Now, to me, a 19- to 20-year-old coming to rehab just doesn't feel right. I know when I was that age, I wouldn't have had enough life experiences to start and complete the 12-step program. No way...

As Christmas 2024 approaches, I'm witnessing a dazzling array of holiday lights illuminating the homes in Uptown New Orleans during my home health visits, though not all of what I encounter is festive. The rehab facility, too, has seen its share of holiday chaos. Reports suggest some patients have been engaging in the illicit trade of medications, prompting the facility to impose restrictions reminiscent of grade school punishments—an attempt to curb juvenile behavior among grown adults. It's disheartening to see rehab patients succumb to a "street" mentality, bartering or selling whatever they can to get by. Many of these individuals, trapped in the throes of addiction, revert to desperate tactics. The old instincts die hard, even amid recovery efforts. Hoarding or dealing pills is, of course, decidedly off-limits. Unfortunately, the entire patient population now faces restrictions: no cell phones, no television, no outside meetings, mandatory book work—it's like a week-long time-out for a room full of riled individuals! The message was clearly meant to be sent. Whispers around the facility hinted that the offenders included both the naïve young patients and the tougher ones marked by past criminal records. A couple of days later, I encountered the patient who had shared tales of potently stealing copper from Charity Hospital; we revisited the topic of the current restrictions. As we talked, he unraveled a wild series of events that vividly played out in my mind like a scene from a gripping drama.

"Yeah G… there was a bunch of us living in the building across from HOD (House of Detention which is now also closed and the one I referenced earlier with the attached video) and there was a dude who fell 9 stories and was still alive…"

I'm sure I had a look of disbelief on my face as I responded…

"No way! Nine stories...? That doesn't seem possible… How was he still alive??

With conviction, he responded…

"Bro… I'm telling you… He was obviously screaming in pain, but I knew not to touch him or try to move him… He looked like a pretzel lying on the ground. There was a few of us who wanted to call an ambulance, and some others didn't, as they felt like they would lose their spot in here…"

At that point, I really didn't know what to say, as I was imagining a bunch of tweakers and homeless drug addicts just lying around in an abandoned prison building with trash, needles, and filth everywhere. He would also go on to tell me how they would get the elevator cable cords and rip them open, as there is a lot of copper in them. He would then go on to tell me more about this, and the story got even crazier…

"Yeah G… the dude was just lying there for hours, and I left to go scrap some copper, and when I came back, he was dead by the time the ambulance arrived… I heard he was begging for a "hot shot" and that may have done him in before the fall… I heard just about every bone in his body was shattered…"

As you might imagine, I was just listening to this in amazement. The fact that someone could fall that far and live is unbelievable, and to do that in that environment and lay there for more than 24 hours is insane! From there, the story gets even wilder.

"Yeah… the police eventually came there to check out the scene, but from what I heard, nothing was even investigated. There was even some lady who had a son who was strung out on drugs, and her son had been missing for some time and was around asking questions… To this day, I have never heard of any formal investigation into it… It was even rumored that he may have been pushed down the elevator shaft and didn't 'fall…'"

Wow… I'm just taking this all in as he tells the story like it was no big deal and said he had plenty of other crazy stories if I ever wanted to hear them. The next day, he was telling me about this story (https://youtu.be/5TNFeAmzaQ0?si=lvWOMe6RZamjKU7A) and I decided to investigate both and was able to confirm this story as another person fell to their death in a now basically abandoned high-rise. He said he was there scrapping copper and getting high when this one happened. Apparently, a fire was started, and smoke quickly consumed the area where this guy was, and he fell or maybe jumped to his death. I couldn't find any info on the first story, but I believe him. The way he told the story and what subsequently transpired totally fit in line with what he told me. Some of the stories of where these people were and how they were living before coming to rehab are quite remarkable.

I decided to work on Christmas Eve for a few hours and Christmas Day as it was a double time/Holiday pay day. The extra cheese is always nice, lol. There happened to be an AA meeting that evening in-house with a special presentation, which was different. Lucky for me, I got a bonus story on this Christmas Day, so it was a win/win.

A recent graduate of the rehab program, I would say about three months ago—before the last hurricane for sure. He strolled into the med room, requesting a couple of Tylenols for a headache, and we exchanged some pleasantries. I asked him how he was doing, and he proceeded to tell me…

"Man, the $200 a month that I have to pay for drug court is making it hard for me to get ahead…"

Of course, I was intrigued now and had to hear the rest of this situation…

"Damn… how long do you have to pay that and why?

"I'm in an 18-month drug court program… After graduating the program here, I entered into an arrangement with the court system to have the drug and burglary charges on me expunged… "

I have to say, I have never heard of this so I can only assume that he was a first-time offender, but I wasn't sure.

'Wow man… I know $200 a month is tough for you, but having the opportunity to have drug and burglary charges expunged is worth it… Just curious… what did you do?"

I could see he was a little down about the situation by the tone of his voice…

"Yeah doc... I was pretty bad off on meth… I broke into a barber shop and a couple of other businesses looking for cash or whatever I could get to pay for the drugs… I finally got caught and arrested…. Was a blessing, really… That shit is deadly… Ruined my life, but I'm working my way back. I'm so glad I'm doing better now..."

Multiple felony charges. I had to investigate, and this is what I found out.

Updated Louisiana expungement laws as of 2020. Not sure if this had anything to do with Covid but here you go:

As of 2019:

During the summer of 2019, the Louisiana legislature made some changes to the existing expungement laws. These changes, which became effective on August 1, 2019, include the following:

Bench warrants

When an expungement order is signed by a judge, the records must be removed from public access. This includes not only the record of arrest and warrants, but also any bench warrant- a warrant issued when the accused fails to appear in court. Bench warrants can be treated like any other warrants, and police use them to bring the defendants back to the courtroom. In the past, people who expunged their records from public access still dealt with records of their bench warrants, but with the new change to the law, this issue has been resolved.

Felony convictions

The legislature also made changes to allow more individuals with felony convictions access to expungement if:

> The prosecution was dismissed; or more than ten years have elapsed since the person completed any sentence or probation for their felony conviction, and the convicted person has not been convicted of any other charge since then. However, the felony charge cannot be expunged if it was a violent or a sex offense crime.

Here are the changes to the LME (Law for Misdemeanor Expungement):

There have been a couple of subtle changes to the law regarding misdemeanor expungements.

If you are charged with a misdemeanor:

> You are eligible for expungement after the prosecution is dismissed or the conviction is set aside as a result of Louisiana Code of Criminal Procedure Article 894(B).
>
> Even if someone did not plead under Article 894(B), they are still eligible for an expungement if five or more years have passed since the sentence was successfully completed.
>
> You are never eligible for an expungement for a sex crime, and one is never eligible for expungement for domestic abuse battery crime.

Changes to the Law for Felony Expungement:

> Some of the changes to the law are specific to felonies because these crimes are more serious and obviously require more stringent standards to complete the expungement.

If you are charged or prosecuted for a felony:

> You are eligible for expungement after the prosecution has dismissed your conviction is set aside as a result of Louisiana Code of Criminal Procedure Article 893(E). Even if you did not plead under Article 893(E), you are eligible for expungement if more than 10 years have passed since your sentence was successfully completed, as long as one has no open felonies charges and/or one has no felony convictions on their record for the 10 years since the completion of one's sentence for the preceding felony.

You are eligible for an expungement if you were convicted of possession of, or possession with intent to distribute, a drug.

You are not eligible for expungement if the crime was for attempted or completed:

Sex Crimes (as it should be)! ***As a caveat to this, there are certain crimes that were defined as sex crimes but are no longer classified this way. If you were convicted or pleaded guilty to one of these crimes, it is possible you are eligible for an expunction of your record. A careful review of your case by an expungement lawyer will be necessary: any domestic abuse or domestic violence crime. There is beginning to be some pushback from the Louisiana State Police, who maintain the Louisiana Bureau of Criminal Identification and Information, who believe that if a defendant was arrested because of a domestic abuse or domestic violence incident, then the defendant is not eligible for an expungement. A skilled expungement attorney should be consulted if your case arose from a domestic disturbance.

A crime of violence pursuant to Louisiana Revised Statute 14:2(B)

A crime involving a minor who is under the age of 17.

One is never eligible for expungement if one is convicted of, or has pleaded guilty to, the distribution or manufacture of any drug or controlled dangerous substance.

***Under the old law, it was unclear whether a person who was in jail could receive an expungement; however, the new law states clearly that expungement for people in prison is not permitted. Additionally, the old law only allowed a person who was convicted or pleaded guilty to a felony was eligible for only one expungement in their entire life. It appears the new law allows for multiple expungements during a defendant's life if it has been greater than 15 years since the last expunction was granted by the court.

There are a few changes to the law in Louisiana regarding expungement that are updated regardless of whether you are convicted of, or plead guilty to, a misdemeanor or a felony. These include:

A Hearing may be held 60 days after a Motion for Expungement is filed.

> At the hearing, the defendants-in-rule (the District Attorney's Office, the Arresting Agency, and the Louisiana State Police) may object to the expunction. They may also waive their objection in writing if they choose. If a party fails to appear for the hearing, fails to file an objection, or fails to waive their appearance in writing, they forfeit their rights to object to the expungement.
>
> This means that there will be a longer turnaround time for an expungement to be completed.

The court costs for most expungements is $500.00 (except for Article 894(B) expungements and pursuant to Article 984)

> $250 will go to the Louisiana Bureau of Criminal Identification and Information.
>
> $50 will go to the arresting agency.
>
> $50 will go to the district attorney where the arrest took place.
>
> $200 will go to the Clerk of Court who shall collect all the fees.
>
> All fees are non-refundable.

Fees may be waived for:

An acquittal or finding of not guilty at trial.

The District Attorney consented to the expungement and the case was dismissed by the District Attorney.

The District Attorney consents to the expungement, the District Attorney's Office refused to prosecute the charges, and the time limit for prosecution of the charges has expired.

The applicant was arrested but not prosecuted within the time limit permitted by law to file a bill of information or obtain a Grand Jury Indictment.

The applicant was found factually innocent because of a post-conviction relief application.

A juvenile who has successfully completed drug court.

During the 2020 Regular Legislative Session, Governor John B. Edwards signed over 330 new bills into law, including several that reference the expungement process.

- **Act 71**

There are certain qualifications that a person must meet in order to be eligible to have an expungement. One requirement in the past has been to qualify for expungement, a person must be employed for ten consecutive years. That is no longer a requirement.

- **Act 79**

There are certain fees that must be paid when filing for expungement. According to the new act, law firms may help their clients make these payments by money order or check. The exact language of the act says, "Payment may be made by United States postal money orders or money orders issued by any state or national bank or by checks issued by a law firm or an attorney."

- **Act 132**

With the signing of this act, someone who was not convicted of a crime, but instead took part in a pretrial diversion program, would now be eligible to file a motion to expunge a record of their arrest.

I hope you find this informative, and you never know who may benefit from this info. We exchanged some more back and forth about his situation all the while I was really getting to see how far a person can fall when battling their addictions.

It was now New Year's Eve and I went in for a couple of hours after my day job to help pass out the evening medications. Come to find out there was an AA party that many of the patients were going to. Interesting… I would think it would be a bit of a challenge for some of these patients to be in a party environment on New Year's Eve. Here's is the invite which was on the Alcoholic's Anonymous New Orleans website (www.aaneworleans.org) and the invite -

(https://aaneworleans.org/event/d20-presents-2025-new-years-eve-paarty/).

I had plans that night, but I slipped away for a little while to go check this out. A New Year's Eve party in New Orleans with no alcohol is different, for sure. I've been to plenty of parties and events with drinking and drugs all around, but never to a party where everyone was an addict and there was no drinking or drugs at all. Interesting!

The next day, I woke up to some horrific news... A terrorist attack on Bourbon St. I was stunned, just watching the television in disbelief. It also dawned on me that I was near that area just a few hours ago on Decatur St. and Jackson Square where some concerts were taking place after the Sugar Bowl parade. Damn... Here is a link to one of the initial reports of this heinous act of pure evil. https://www.cbsnews.com/news/bourbon-street-new-orleans-attack-suspect-what-to-know/ This also shows about where I was on this night and how random things can be.

After spending a significant amount of time absorbing the somber realities broadcast on national news, I found my heart heavy yet reflective. The stretch of Bourbon Street I was reminded of has long been riddled with issues, one I deliberately tend to avoid. This particular night, fresh off work, I ventured to the Roosevelt Hotel, hoping to enjoy drinks with some friends before making my way to a different gathering on Decatur Street, where a concert awaited. As I strolled past the very spot where a terrorist had brazenly maneuvered his truck around the police barricade, I glanced at my watch—around 7:30 p.m. I was faced with two routes: to veer left onto Bourbon, bypassing through a side street toward Jackson Square, or to forge ahead straight to Decatur. I chose the latter. Though it was merely 7:30 p.m. and not the early hours of the morning, I had traversed that part of Bourbon Street countless times. Flanking the road were renowned restaurants bustling with life, making it a hotspot of activity. Unfortunately, that very corner of Canal Street and Bourbon has been the scene of multiple shootings through the years, with Canal Street's proximity to the I-10 Interstate suggesting it's a prime escape route for anyone wishing to flee a dangerous scene.

Anyway, we were down at Jackson Square for a good while, checking out the scene. After a while, we all decided to walk to Caesar's Casino to hang out and people-watch! It was extremely crowded there, as expected, and after we all had a couple of drinks and cowed in on a few football bets (a cow is when a few people put some money together and make some bets with the hope of splitting the winnings - fun way to gamble and not get too crazy). Eventually, there was some talk of walking over to Bourbon St., but it was around 10:30, and I decided to call it a night. In my younger days I would have gone without hesitation. Glad I did. Still can't believe it happened. In my lifetime I've seen terrorist attacks all over the world and many in other places in the US, but to have it happen in my city is still surreal.

With the world changing a rapid pace, an increase in terror attacks around the globe, school shootings, and disgruntled employees attacking and killing former co-workers, I decided to do a little research and provide you with knowledge and information if you are ever confronted with this type of evil.

Here is an active shooter preparation checklist that may save your life and the lives of those close to you. You can use this checklist as a guideline to prepare yourself for running during an active shooter event.

1. Run
    - Be sure to identify the emergency exits or nearest exit points. Identify the two closest exits to where you are in relation to getting out of the building.
    - Be sure to run with intention. Are there any obstructions? Do you have a clear path out? Are you running in the opposite direction from the attacker?
    - Know where you're going? Designate an assembly spot. Identify a 2nd place of safety (be specify).
2. Hide
    - You can use the following checklist as a guide to prepare yourself for hiding during an active shooter event.
    - Hide. If you are unable to run out of the building, quickly and calmly get to a hiding place. How far are you from your hiding spot? Are there any obstructions

in your way? Are you moving away from the attacker? Be sure to have this area predetermined if an event were to take place. Many individuals just freeze from the shock of an event happening like this and understandably so. Being calm under extreme pressure is rare but can be learned. Fight or flight... We have all heard it in our lives. That's basically what's happening here.

- Take cover. If you can do so this will usually be able to withstand a bullet. Is it in a lockable space? This can deter an active shooter if the door is locked and barricaded with something heavy enough to make an active shooter move on. Are there any windows? Avoid windows at all costs if possible. Conceal yourself as much as possible.

3. Fight
    - Get a weapon to defend yourself. A fire extinguisher if possible is good. You can spray the perpetrator in the eyes and/or use it to hit them. If not, then what is the closest item to you to be used to defend yourself? Can you use the object comfortably to defend yourself?
    - The next thing is very important.
    - Fight offensively! Do not wait for the attacker to come to you. Go at them. It could literally be a matter of life and death. What's your plan to take the attacker down? Poke the eyes, punch the windpipe/throat? Pepper spray? Have a plan to attack and stun the attacker before they come at you first.

Next is an example of a workplace Emergency Action Plan Checklist:

An emergency plan should consider an active shooter event occurring at the workplace. We have seen a significant rise in school/workplace shootings in recent times. Silent alarms for intruders, or alerts for smoke, gunfire, or even an explosion, should be considered. An emergency plan should consider the impact an active shooter event could have on everyday workplace operations. Staff members can brainstorm different scenarios and practice to see what works best for them.

Here's something to consider as well. Does the plan contain the names and contact information for individuals responsible for implementation of the plan? The plan should include names, titles, departments, and telephone numbers of people to contact and an explanation of the duties and responsibilities each employee is responsible for. Does the plan accommodate all employees' personal information and emergency contacts? The plan should contain relevant personal information for employees, including their emergency contacts, disabilities, and allergies if possible.

Does the plan contain contact information for local emergency services? The plan should contain updated information on all emergency and rescue services within a particular area or within the district. Something else to consider...

Does the plan accommodate aftercare following an emergency event? The plan should contain information on what to do following an emergency. This would include medical healthcare and mental healthcare. Does the plan accommodate an evacuation protocol? There should be multiple evacuation plans in place for different scenarios. All staff members should be made aware of these plans. This was mentioned in the active shooter scenario as well.

Does the plan identify the relevant assembly points? Assembly points should be allocated and marked. Employees should be given notice of their respective assembly points. Does the plan identify how to alert employees to an emergency? The alarms and detectors should be checked and maintained regularly. Ensure there is a plan in place to calmly alert employees of an emergency.

All of this can be planned for, but there needs to be some live reps to be done... Does the plan allow for regular drills to be conducted? Regular drills of evacuation scenarios should be carried out. There should also be records of when the last drill was conducted, when the next one is scheduled, and any issues that may have come up during the drills.

It's unfortunate that we live in a world where this is even possible, but we do. It's easy to think this could never "happen to me" and I've been guilty of thinking that way, but not anymore. This attack in New Orleans on New Year's Eve has been a wake-up call. Having been near where it happened opened my eyes to how easily that could have been me. After a few days of this horrible event transpiring, the MCC – Metropolitan Crime Commission put out the following article (https://metrocrime.org/as-super-bowl-looms-new-orleans-officials-to-review-security-in-wake-of-deadly-attack/) reviewing what happened and what increased measures will be in place for the Super Bowl which will be played on February 9th 2025. Here is another article about what the family of the terrorist attacker had to say (https://x.com/nolanews/status/1876132916603826220?s=12). Unreal…

In the days leading up to the Super Bowl the city was buzzing with excitement, and you could see and feel a bigger police and military presence. The terrorist attack was still being talked about as the big weekend was finally here.

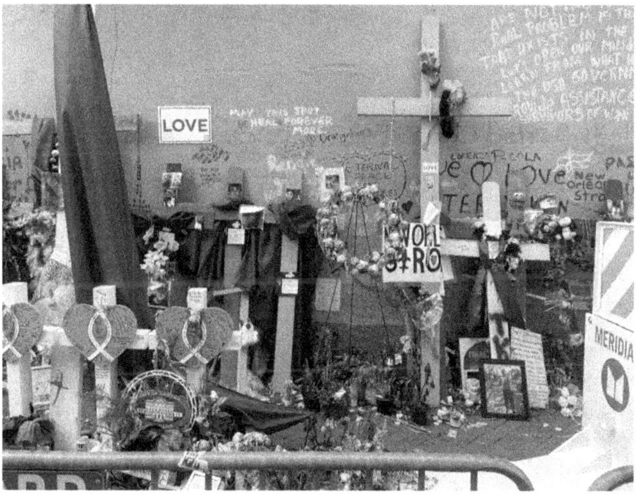

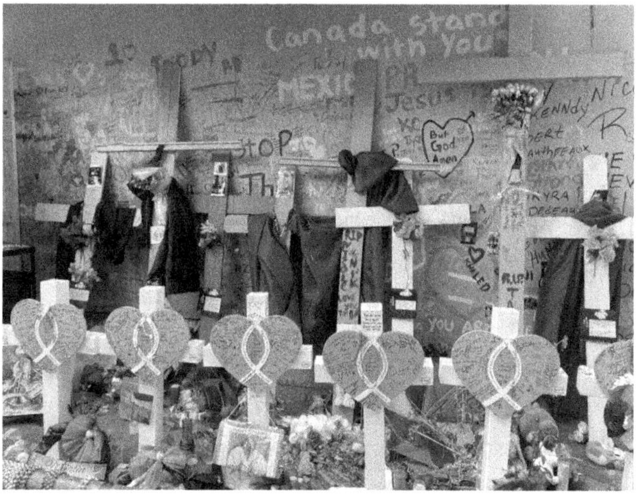

I went to a pre-Super Bowl party downtown in the Warehouse District of New Orleans and saw a former patient there from the rehab. I didn't want to go say hello in case they might feel uncomfortable, so I kind of slid back and figured if they came up to me and said hi, that would be ok. The party was cool, with some former NFL'er and a few celebrities there. A few of us walked over to Caesar's afterward, and there was a vast amount of security around. Here are some things to check out in regards to the terror attack and the superbowl.

www.fbi.gov/bourbonstreetupdates,

dLIwu7wapcxW2r_FQ==&ch=ZOpDML9xQukIpMjUp-D-7F74CpaS-DrEDrH31PHOGjqg3fvkwW-srg=="ch=ZOpDML9xQukIpMjUp-D-7F74CpaS-DrEDr-H31PHOGjqg3fvkwW-srg=="bourbonstreetvictims

As the New Year unfolds at the Rehab, the Prison, and the Home Health, the varied narratives woven through the lives of these individuals are quite interesting! At the rehab center, local medical students in the first year of their training run a free clinic each week, where they undertake to create medical histories and conduct physical examinations for newly admitted patients. Guided by a professor, this initiative serves a dual purpose: it sharpens the students' clinical skills while simultaneously providing invaluable medical assistance to the residents. Following a brief hiatus for the holidays, the clinic resumed operations just a week after the tragic Bourbon St terror attack, highlighting a community's resilience and the intertwined fates of healers and those in need.

A couple of days into the new year, I was talking to one of the patients during an evening medication pass, and we got to discussing the terror attack. This patient said, "Did you hear about… In 2004 he was in the Tsunami in Indonesia… He said one second he was in his hotel room, and the next he was pulled out of the window of his room and was clinging to a tree in the water while people were getting sucked out to sea…"

I immediately could visualize this and remember the images that were on tv when the Tsunami hit. 180,000+ died I believe... Incredible...

"Wow... that's insane! How long did he have to cling to that tree?"

The patient didn't know but talked about all the people he said were getting sucked back out to sea... "The screaming and chaos were deafening," he said... I can only imagine..."

Taking this all in, it reminds me of all the tragic events that have taken place in the last 20 years... 9-11, was probably the start of it and since then the Gulf Wars, the 2004 Tsunami, Katrina, the BP oil spill, multiple terror attacks, theCovid Pandemic... The world is on fire as predicted in Revelation and this is just the beginning of sorrows...we are indeed living in the End Times. On a funnier note, I acquired a new nickname!

The next day, I was passing the meds out at approximately 9:30 pm and one of the younger patients strolls into the med room and blurts out "what's up Rehab Dad!" It took me a second to process what he said, and I let out a little laugh.

"Funny! When did you come up with that one?"

The patient was probably in his mid-twenties and a good-looking fella with a couple of piercings and tattoos.

"Yeah doc... a couple of the other nurses said that we kind of looked alike, so I came up with Rehab Dad!"

I guess I can see it, but damn, I guess I could be this dude's dad, lol. My dadlol. My dad had me at 50 years old and I don't have kids so I never really think about the fact that I could technically even be a grandpa! Geez... Oh well guess I have a new nickname at the rehab. Will see if it sticks...

It is now mid-January, and the city has been hit by a historic snowstorm. Here is a little funny fact from Twitter or X or whatever they call it -https://x.com/nwsanchorage/status/1882082172057899062?s=12.

The pictures that emerged from the snowstorm, especially of some of New Orleans' most iconic places, were truly amazing! I can't imagine ever seeing snow like that again.

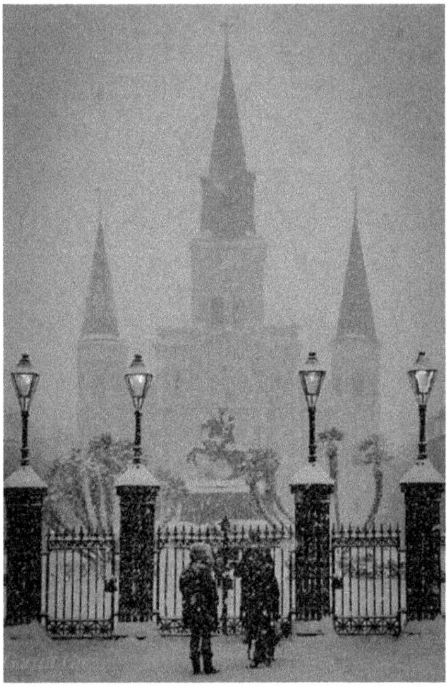

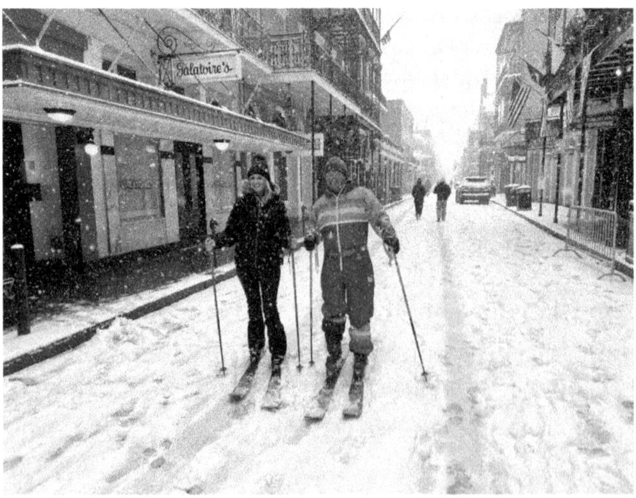

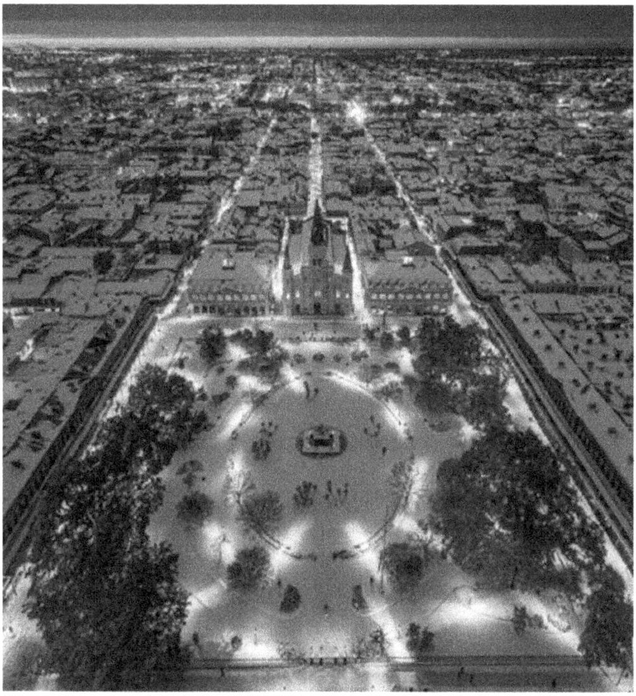

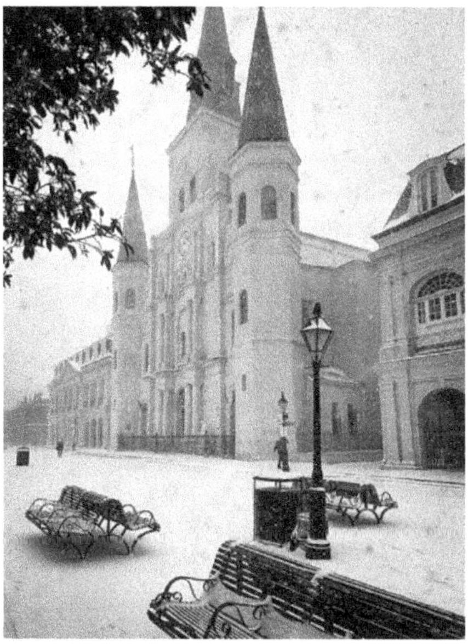

The city was buzzing with the Super Bowl about a week away. The city was getting rave reviews for all the great food, drinks, sights, and sounds. The SEAR 1 terrorism designation and all that went with it brought an interesting element to the city. I heard about the terror attack memorial at the beginning of Bourbon St. and decided to go look at it. It was somber to see. I had never seen anything quite like that. When my brother passed away, there was a similar memorial that many of his friends created near where they found him in the water. He did two tours of duty in Iraq, survived a tank attack while saving a couple of his fellow servicemen, earning a Gold Star, was honorably discharged from the Army, and never really could adjust to life afterward. Unfortunately, he was found face down in an area of water where he used to hang out with his friends in high school in Waveland, Mississippi. They think he may have had a seizure, and he did suffer a Traumatic Brain Injury while fighting in Iraq... RIP my brother.

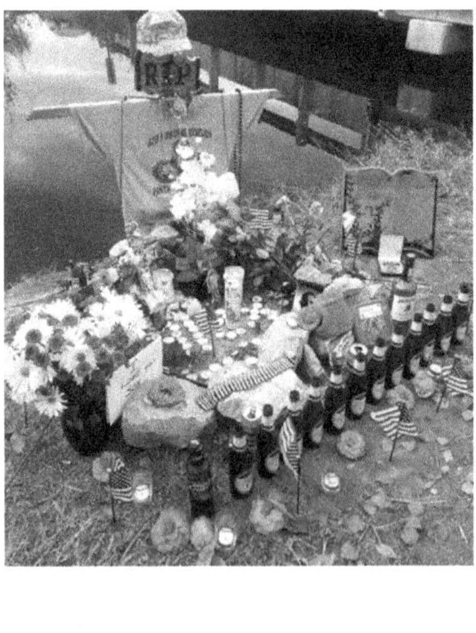

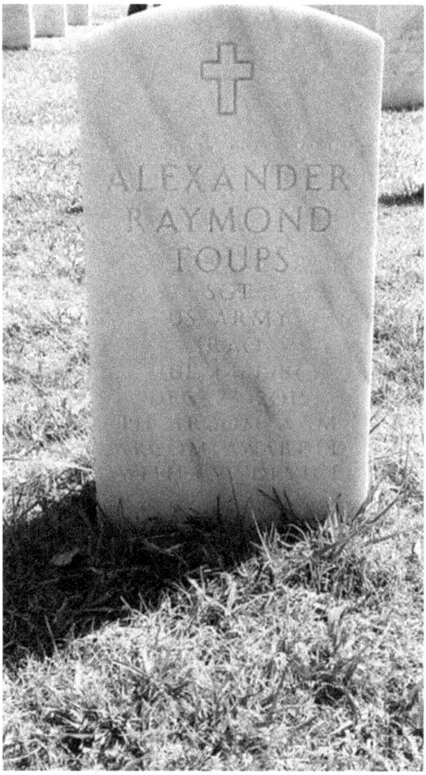

The Super Bowl was a resounding success, and the city of New Orleans shone brightly on the global stage, especially with Mardi Gras just around the corner. After the tragic events of the January 1st, 2025, terror attack, the city showcased an impressive comeback. Some patients managed to work at the Super Bowl, and they even enjoyed the game for free! I heard tickets were selling for over $5,000—a staggering sum, but if someone has the means, why not indulge a little?

The SEAR 1 terror designation lingered in the air, a palpable presence during the festivities. Mardi Gras thrived, with the final crime statistics reflecting an impressive decline—no significant incidents to report. Sure, the weather played tricks, shifting some parades to different days, but that's part of the charm. Yet, it felt peculiar to witness such a heightened security presence throughout the revelry.

I hope you found this part of the journey through a city steeped in color and history enjoyable. This corner of the world is quite distinctive, with its shadowy tales now surfacing. I trust this part of the narrative is entertaining, enlightening, humorous, and thought-provoking. For further exploration, check out this website I stumbled upon during my research: www.drugfreeworld.com. It's a comprehensive A to Z reference and educational guide covering drug programs, interactive applications, real stories from real people, and documentaries that reveal the truth about drugs. Truly fascinating.

Now I'm going to take you back in time to an incredible story of survival in an unimaginable situation—how I ended up here some 20 years ago…

8 inmates still on the run after Orleans jail escape; sheriff cites lock failures One escapee has been recaptured. OPSO confirms security failures, potential inside assistance, and infrastructure problems at the jail.
https://www.wwltv.com/mobile/article/news/local/orleans-parish-jail-lockdown-inmate-escape-may-2025/289-5716dc35-cc62-4c1e-b29b-d1ef72ad5532

'I found out from my mother': Victim speaks out after New Orleans jailbreak as fear ripples through community A shooting survivor criticizes system failures after learning about his attacker's prison escape via a relative instead of official channels.
https://www.wwltv.com/mobile/article/news/crime/new-orleans-jail-escape/i-should-have-been-the-first-on-the-list-victim-says-he-wasnt-warned-after-escape/289-e448d935-2942-4d71-8662-6cf5f78c83df

Part Two

Chapter 8

The Prison

Orleans Parish Prison, in the center of New Orleans, is one of the most notorious jails in the United States. It regularly houses over 6,000 prisoners and has a documented history of being one of the roughest, toughest prisons in the country.

After Katrina hit and the levees broke, electric power went out, and the prison complex was thrust into darkness. Floodwaters swamped restless prisoners in locked cells; some were left in chest-high contaminated waters. Inmates were trapped with little food or water, and prison guards were ordered to stay at their posts. Some left their posts and many employees, including doctors, nurses and others, had to fend for themselves.

It was a hot, hellish week I will never, ever forget. I pleaded with my 83-year-old father to evacuate but he refused. I was only 33, and I had recently accepted the fact I had to look after him a little more. I never imagined I would have to keep him alive under those unimaginable conditions and circumstances though.

Midnight was upon us, and it was starting to get pretty quiet. Hurricane Katrina was swirling angrily off the Gulf Coast from Texas to Florida and would make landfall soon. And it was headed straight for New Orleans.

I could hear the gusting winds outside and by this point, the lights around the city were flickering out. I was on the 10th floor of the House of Detention (HOD) finishing my shift and was able to get a good look outside. It was a light show to say the least.

Transformers were blowing up, shooting sparks. When they exploded, they gave off a purplish-white light and sizzled like colossal sparklers. Amazingly, I could see an occasional car traveling on the road as the rain came down and entire areas of the city started to go dark. Billboard signs blew away, and our building started slightly swaying from nature's forces. It was beginning to get daunting ... and scary. After about an hour of watching the city slide into what I would later learn was a true disaster, I decided I better try to get some rest in preparation for work the next day.

I took the stairwell downstairs; the lights were flashing and fading all the way down, and then they went completely out. It was like being in a cave. I waited a minute, but the lights didn't come back on. I was between the seventh and eighth floors of the prison and could hear some inmates yelling and rattling bars of their cages. I'm sure they were somewhat frightened. I was nervous, and I wasn't in a cell. Feeling for the handrails, I walked slowly down the stairs into more darkness.

It was eerie.

Thankfully, when I got to the second floor, the back-up generator cranked up, and the lights came back on. I decided to lie down on my makeshift bed and get some sleep. The last thing I remember that night was hearing scattered radios blaring bleak messages in a sinister stereo. I could hear the fear in everyone's voices as a somber mood overtook the City. Those around me appeared to realize that it was going to be bad. Real bad. I took one more look at my sleeping father, said a few prayers, and went to sleep.

Tossing and turning all night, I got maybe four or five hours of sleep between unsettling waking moments. That would be the last bit of sleep I would get for what seemed like days. A touch of rainy, cloudy daylight crept in through the a window. My dad started to wake up and sheepishly asked where the showers were.

Laughing to myself, I said, "Showers? Not here, Dad. We could go into the bathroom and use the sink to wet a rag or towel if you want."

Looking agitated, he said, "No, that's all right. I just have to take my pills."

"Help yourself," I said.

The bathrooms still worked at this point, so after he took his pills, we went the break room to get some breakfast.

"What's up Will?" I said to the deputy.

"Nuttin', Gavin. What's up with you?" Will, a young, husky African-American, had worked at the jail probably as long as I had.

"Just comin' to see what's for breakfast," I said.

Smiling, he said, "Oh you know, we got those runny scrambled eggs, soupy oatmeal, and some dry-ass jail biscuits!"

"Sounds good. Can I get some for me and my dad?"

"That's your dad? What's up, Pops?"

"Hey, how y'all doin'?" my dad replied.

"Can't complain. You're son's a cool mo fo. Ya heard me, Pops?"

My dad turned to me with an of, *What the hell did he just say?*

A second or two later, it must have hit him. "Oh yeah... thanks. He's a good son," my dad finally responded.

"Let me scoop y'all up some of this wonderful IHOP real quick!" Deputy Will joked.

"Thanks Will."

As we got our food, we tried to find an open area to sit and eat. Looking out the steel-mesh-barred window, the water level in the street didn't look that bad, maybe a foot or two high. Seasoned New Orleanians had seen more than that accumulate from a routine heavy rain. It was coming down in sheets, and the wind had kicked up. The good news was the water level was nowhere near my dad's car nor mine, and I was starting to think we might get lucky.

"Hey Son, can you get some salt or something? This tastes like crap!"

I had to laugh. "Yeah. Let me see what I can find. I told you that you should have left with Gladys and Norman (my aunt and uncle). You're eating prison food now."

"Just get me some salt, Son. I don't want to hear all that!"

"Calm down. Calm down. I'll find you something." The area was really crowded, but there was no problem finding salt. "Here you go. Bon appétit."

"Bone what?" my dad asked, confused.

"Never mind. Enjoy your breakfast."

Afterward, he decided to stay and watch TV, and I went up to the 10th floor to take a look at the city. The 10th floor is just high enough to get an expansive 360-degree view – except that some of the view is obstructed by the small, reinforced windows.

As I stepped into the elevator, I noticed the floor was wet. The only other time I saw the elevator in this condition was when one of our inmates got the brilliant idea to jump up and pull on a sprinkler system pipe that runs down the tier. It caused the water to explode out of the pipes and run down the elevator shaft, flooding the first two floors of the building.

When I got off the elevator on the 10th floor it had a few inches of water on it. Going to into the psych office, it looked like a tornado had demolished it. There was a big wooden board covering the hole where the air conditioning unit was. At about 5 a.m., the wind had blown the unit into the office and over the desk by the window. Nurse Donna was sitting in the middle of the mess.

Donna is a middle-aged black woman. She had worked at the jail off and on for over 12 years primarily as a psych nurse. She also has a mouth like a sailor. Donna had been resting her feet on the desk when the blustery winds blew the air conditioning unit into the psych office and nearly knocked her on the floor.

"Gavin, you should have seen that shit! That unit came flyin', and then the rain followed right behind it," Donna said. "You all right? You look a little wet."

"Ha ha, smart ass. Of course I'm wet. The rain was flying all over the place. We were trying to cover the opening up with anything we could get our hands on."

In the office, the copy machine, computers, psych papers, and various other things were either wet or scattered on the ground. At one point, Donna and Nurse Robert said they had to get out of the office because the wind and rain were too strong.

"Man, I slipped and fell on my ass and everything! You should have seen it!" Donna said.

"I would have paid big money to see that!"

"Screw you, Gavin! Screw you." She laughed about it and talked about what went on the night before.

Around 11 a.m., the weather outside appeared to be improving. Looking out one of the second-floor windows, the damage around our building didn't look that bad. The water level outside appeared to be between two and three feet, and it seemed we were through most of the storm. I was thinking maybe we had made out okay.

Lunchtime was approaching, and I went to check on my dad. He was lying down, listening to the radio and reading a magazine. I asked him what he was reading and he said, "This is some kind of fashion magazine."

I was a little surprised, "Where did you get that?"

With a guilty look on his face, he pointed to his right and said, "Out of that bag over there."

I turned to see what he was talking about, and about 15 feet from us was an open school bag.

A little stunned, I asked, "Did you take that out of there, Dad?"

"Yeah, why?"

"You can't go looking through other people's stuff! You tryin' to get me in trouble or what?"

"No, don't worry. I was gonna put it back."

"Come on, Dad. Don't go looking in other people's stuff like that! You might really piss someone off. I don't need that right now. You're not at home."

"All right, all right. I'll put it back."

"Hurry up. Better yet, give it here and I'll do it." Now I knew my dad must really be bored to go looking through the bag of someone he doesn't even know — and reading a fashion magazine.

It made me think back to a story that gets told every year at my Aunt Gladys and Uncle Norman's house during Christmas dinner. Both my dad and my uncle were in World War II in Reims, France. Both men were musicians, but my dad was in the Army band, and my uncle was fighting in the war. My dad played saxophone and clarinet, and my uncle played trumpet. They didn't know each other until one fateful day when my dad sat on my Uncle Norman's bunk and was looking through Norman's mail.

Enraged, Norman asked, "What the hell are you doing?"

My dad, just being his usual self said, "You're from New Orleans? So am I!"

As the story goes, Uncle Norman shot back, "What the hell does that have to do with you looking through my mail?"

"I have a sister back in New Orleans who I'd like to set you up with when you get back home."

Norman says he immediately thought to himself, *Great; this guy's trying to set me up with his fat, ugly sister.* He did agree to meet my dad's sister, and when he went to the door to pick her up he was amazed to see how beautiful she was.

"Gavin let me tell you, your Aunt Gladys had the most beautiful tanned body I had ever seen and it was LOVE at first sight!" And they have been together ever since. They recently celebrated their 60th wedding anniversary.

That's a glimpse into the mind of my dear old dad.

At about 3:15 p.m., I went up to the 10th floor to go to work, performing my nursing duties. I told my dad I'd see him later and to stay out of trouble. I felt funny saying that because it was like warning a kid or something. When I got to the 10th floor, I got a report from the day nurse, and that's when the fun really started. One of our "regular" arrestees, J.W., had hurt himself.

He's a white male, about 30 years old, with a multitude of psychiatric illnesses. I really can't completely describe J.W., but I'll try. He is, by far, the most bizarre, out-of-touch with reality person with whom I have ever come in contact. No one knows where he is from or if he has any family. He's thin and stands about five feet, eight inches tall. He's missing his two front teeth, has greasy light brown hair and pasty white skin, and he speaks with an accent like a 10-year-old country boy.

J.W. has multiple personalities: One day he thinks he's Elvis Presley, and the next day he is calling me "Dad" or saying, "Hey Jim, you're my brother." Sometimes he thinks he's Kurt Cobain, and at other times he thinks he's George W. Bush.

J.W. was on the floor that day, playing in the water that had come in when the air conditioning unit blew into the office. While frolicking, he slipped and hit his head on his cell's toilet, cutting his skull wide open. It required a dozen stitches to close.

The doctor ordered "neuro checks Q1 X 24." That meant we had to check his vital signs every hour and make sure his eyes would properly react to light. We also were to ask him some basic questions, like his name and the date, even the name of the current president of the United States. With his mental condition, J.W. might say anything on any given day, so this part of the test wasn't much good.

The first check was all right, but during the second one J.W. looked really pale and said, "I'm real dizzy." His blood pressure was dangerously low, and his pulse was racing. Both were potentially very risky and demanded immediate attention, especially the blood pressure. I notified the doctor on call at one of the other facilities, and he ordered a saline water I.V. to pump fluid directly into J.W.'s veins in order to bring up his blood pressure and lower his pulse rate — STAT. The main problem was we were dealing with a psychiatric inmate who lacked reason, common sense, and a normal understanding of reality. He might not understand we were trying to help him with the treatment.

Having dealt with J.W. on a regular basis for the past few years, I had developed a pretty good rapport with him.

"Hey Dad, I don't feel good ... I think I'm gonna pass out," he said to me.

"J.W., when was the last time you ate or drank anything?" I asked.

"I don't know, but I'm hungry, Dad."

"All right, J.W., can you walk up to the front so I can get you something to drink?"

"Sure thing, Daddy!"

I walked briskly to the back storage room, making sure not to slip and fall, and I got a PowerAde drink for him out of the refrigerator.

"Hold still, all right? I need to start an I.V. on you."

As he began to drink the PowerAde, I went to the medical supply room to get the needed intravenous supplies.

"Why are you doing that, Dad?"

"J.W., I'm not your dad. Now sit still."

"Don't say that, Dad, please. What are you doing? Don't! That hurts!"

"J.W., sit still and shut up!"

At this point, I could see that this was going to be a problem, and I called the second floor to get another nurse to help me. In addition to dealing with this situation, I could hear the rest of the inmates on the floor yelling for food, medications, and demanding to change the channel on the television. The storm was picking back up, and the atmosphere was getting frenzied.

After a few minutes, Nurse Urban showed up, to my relief.

"What seems to be the problem?" he asked.

"J.W.'s blood pressure is about 50/30 and his pulse is quite elevated. I called the doctor and he wants an I.V. STAT. He keeps moving all over the damn place."

We convinced J.W. to lie down on a bench to help restrict his movement.

"Hey Gavin, hold his shoulder down while I try his other arm."

"Dad, what the hell are y'all doin'? That hurts. Stop!"

As we were tending to him and I was trying to explain that I was helping him, I looked down the tier and saw two inmates fighting.

"Hang on a second. Let me go get some deputies to break up that fight in the back!" I said. I was hoping Nurse Urban would be able to calm J.W. while I was gone.

Running down the central walkway, I slipped on some water and almost fell flat on my butt. I was able to catch the door and regain my balance before I fell in all the water. After notifying Security of the fight, I returned to try and get the I.V. started.

Checking his blood pressure again, I couldn't get a diastolic reading.

This was about to be a critical situation. Although J.W. didn't know it, and I couldn't explain it to him, his condition was life-threatening. Normally when someone is in a condition this bad, we would route him or her to a hospital by ambulance, but that was not an option. With the streets flooded and the storm raging, we had to make do. Even though he was not a typical and contributing member of society, it was our job as nurses and employees of the Criminal Sheriff's Office to do everything we could for him as we would do for anyone with a health problem.

"Stop now! I can't take it anymore!" J.W. screamed.

With our frustration mounting, we decided to take a break.

In his country boy twang, J.W. said, "Thanks Dad. Please don't do that anymore."

"Listen, J.W., just stay still, lie down, and keep quiet. Got it?"

I told Urban we should get a couple of the other nurses up there to give us a hand. At this point, the fight I mentioned had resulted in one of the inmates having a cut above his right eye that also needed stitches.

"Call Dr. Marcus and let him know that we've got someone else who needs stitches," I told Urban.

"Don't you remember? The doctors are all in other buildings," he replied. "We have none here."

"Oh, man! You gotta be kidding." I cleaned and covered the inmate's cut until he could see a doctor.

"Hey, I'm going to get a couple of nurses to help us," I said.

As I made my way to the elevator, I could hear the females in the psychiatric ward whooping and hollering for their medicines.

"Hey all you mother fuckin' nurses and deputies, give us our damn medicine!" a female prisoner yelled. To make matters worse, the disciplinary females were on the opposite side of the psych females, egging them on.

"Y'all bitches are gonna die up in here!"

"Yeah, that's right!"

The situation was getting ugly real quick. It seemed like an eternity while I waited for the elevator, and then I heard a voice over the intercom, "Hey Gavin, the elevator ain't working. You're gonna have to take the stairs."

Making my way to the stairwell, I looked out the window and could see three buildings in Mid-City ablaze. I did have some hope when I saw piece of the sun showing itself behind the clouds. It appeared the storm was just about over.

The sun hadn't even set when the sound of gunfire began crackling off in the distance. I didn't know what was going on, who was doing the shooting, or where it was coming from. But once they started, I didn't think they would stop. I jumped at each of them. They were sporadic and seemed to be ringing out in every direction in the city.

I turned my attention back to my duties and tried to ignore the chilling gunfire. I made my way down the eight flights of stairs to the second floor to get some help with J.W. After locating two available nurses, I said, "Hey, can y'all come up to the 10th floor and help us with an I.V.? We're gonna have to hold him down while y'all try to stick him. The only problem is the elevator isn't working right now. We gotta take the stairs."

They reluctantly agreed. "I'm gonna go check on my dad real quick, and then I'll be up there. Nurse Urban is already up there tryin' to keep J.W. calm," I explained to them. Then I left and made my way over to the little spot on the second floor where my dad and I were camped out.

"Hey Dad, what's up?" I could see he wasn't happy.

"What's up? Oh, I don't know. You tell me." It was obvious he was aggravated by the situation, but there was nothing I could do.

"I bet you wish you would have left, huh?"

"No kidding, Son."

"Hey, you don't have to get short with me. I told you to leave."

"Yeah, I know. I just want to take a shower!"

"That makes two of us. Hey, did you get something to eat? I got some canned goods if you want to heat something up in the microwave," I said, pointing toward the break room.

"What do you have?"

"Take a look in that little green bag right there." I asked one of the other nurses' mothers if she wouldn't mind taking my dad to the break room to help him heat his food. I needed to quickly get back to J.W. I took the stairs back to the 10th floor to see what we could do with our patient, stopping on the eighth floor to catch my breath. Along the way, I could hear the rattling of the bars and menacing chants from the inmates. Once I got to the 10th floor and made a turn off the stairwell, there was a nurse sitting on the floor getting medical assistance.

"What the hell happened?"

Evidently, she had asthma and had aggravated her condition by taking the stairs from the second floor to the 10th floor. As if she was on her last breath, she struggled to say, "I'm ... hum ... gonna, gonna ... be ... all ... all ... all right."

Right behind her, J.W. saw me and said, "Hey Dad. You back? Where you been?"

I replied, "Hey, Son, I'm here. You being a good boy?"

Everyone began to laugh, putting the bizarre and deteriorating situation on hold.

"Yeah, Dad. Can I have something to eat? I'm starving."

"After we get this I.V. started you can eat."

"No, dammit! I want to eat now."

"Well, Son, you're gonna have to wait a little longer." I heard a few more chuckles from the background.

He lunged at me, "Goddammit, I want to eat!"

"You better sit the hell down now! Now! Now, J.W. Now!" I shouted.

Urban grabbed him from behind with a full-nelson move and sat him on the bench. After a minute or two of calming him down, we took some more vital signs; they were still not good.

His blood pressure was still dangerously low, and his heart was beating dangerously hard. He appeared all right and feisty on the outside, but internally, he was in a lot of trouble.

With his vital signs at those levels for any length of time, he could go into heart failure and die. Nurse Yolanda was starting to catch her breath and said, "Y'all stand back. Let me see if I can start an I.V. on this crazy sonofabitch!"

In a joking manner, I jumped back and told J.W., "Look, you done pissed off your mother now. You're gonna be grounded!"

It was perhaps odd that on the brink of our first possible fatality, I tried to find a second or two to lighten the mood; but truly, we were all focused on saving his life.

The nurse said, "Hold him still; give me a 20-gauge needle. Gavin, hold his feet and legs still and you, Favis, get that line ready to go."

J.W.'s eyes got real wide and a look of terror overcame his face. "What the hell are y'all doin' to me? No! Stop! No!" The toughest part was the fact that since J.W. is crazy — literally — we could not reason with him and make him understand we were trying to save his life.

"Listen J.W., please work with us," I said. "Be still and calm. We are trying to help you. Your life is in danger."

"No! Stop! Gimmie somethin' to eat!"

"Fuck it! Hold him still ... I'm going to stick him!" With that, my asthmatic colleague tried five different veins with no success. All the while, J.W. screamed and cried like a 10-year-old child. After about 15 minutes J.W.'s arms looked like pincushions, so we decided to call the medical director to see what he wanted told do. Charity Hospital is about a mile from our building, and by that time, we were surrounded by about four to six feet of water.

Although the weather was clearing, it was still unsafe out there. We had no way of knowing Charity was barely functioning, and wouldn't have been able to help anyway.

After getting word to the medical director through a deputy, and then a ranking official, we were told to bring J.W. to the second floor and he was going to swim over — yes, swim — from IPC (Intake Processing Center). I heard from a couple of deputies they tried to build a dam near the entrance to our building, but those attempts were unsuccessful.

"I'll be there as soon as I can. Try to calm him down and take his vital signs every five minutes until I get there," the medical director said. A deputy was called to the medical office and asked to secure J.W. so we could bring him to the second floor via the stairwell. As we were getting ready to go someone asked sarcastically, "Where are we bringing Elvis? To Graceland or what?"

Again, we had a few laughs. J.W. innocently asked, "We goin' home, Dad?"

At this point, I wanted to keep him as calm as possible, so I replied, "If you're a good boy we might. Just cooperate with us, and we'll see."

"That's great, Dad! I'll be good, I promise. I Promise!"

And with that, we handcuffed J.W. and slowly walked him down the hot, muggy, stairwell — carefully, *very* carefully.

Chapter 9

The Storm

By now it was about 8 p.m. or so, and I hadn't talked to my dad in a while. I asked another nurse to stay with J.W. for a few minutes so I could check on him. After going to the break room and finding the television not working, I went to the west side of the second floor to see who was over there.

I surveyed the area and asked, "Anybody seen my dad?"

A couple deputies said he was over on the south side listening to the radio with some other families.

While heading that way, I overheard someone say the storm completely demolished the Twin Span bridges. Those bridges, each about five miles long, connect eastern New Orleans to the suburb of Slidell across a narrow section of Lake Pontchartrain. The "Twin Spans," as locals call them, are a vital link between the city and eastern and northern suburbs. I couldn't believe it. Entire sections of the bridges just plain gone. If the destruction I was hearing about was true, I wondered if other bridges throughout the city were damaged as well.

When I found my dad, he was playing cards with three deputies and a couple other guys. After a few moments of taking in this scene, I softly asked, "What's up, Dad?"

Looking a bit surprised to see me, he said, "Uh ... just playing cards and listening to the radio, Son."

"Did you eat any dinner?"

"Yeah, I had some kind of stew with chicken in it ... it was okay."

"You been taking your medicine?" I asked.

"Oh yes, Son! I only have about five blood pressure pills left," he said while lighting up a cigarette.

"I'll go upstairs later and see if we have any. We have someone who's sick who we're tryin' to take care of. I'll talk to you later."

"All right, Son. See you later."

As I started to walk away, the deputies said, "We'll keep an eye on him." I thanked them and went back to my duties. I hoped Dad wasn't playing cards for any money, although money wouldn't have done him any good in there. Walking back toward the second floor clinic, I spotted Dr. Inglese trying to dry off with paper towels. With a little smile, I asked, "A little wet out there, huh?"

"Just a little, Gavin. Where's J.W.?"

"He should be in the back room of the second floor clinic. He thinks he's going back to Graceland."

With a puzzled look he asked, "What? Why would he think that?" Obviously, he was not too familiar with J.W.'s personality and with six or seven thousand inmates, why would he be?

"Well, today he thinks he's Elvis Presley. Tomorrow, if there is a tomorrow for him, he might be Kurt Cobain. You never know with J.W."

Smiling sternly, Dr. Inglese said, "Now Gavin, you know you're not supposed to acknowledge things like that with a mentally ill person."

"I know, but the situation was becoming very chaotic and he seemed to calm down a little when the subject of Graceland came up."

"How the hell did that come up anyway?" the doctor asked.

"Please, don't ask. Let's just go and see how he is."

The second floor clinic is a room with a few desks, computers, no air conditioning even on a normal day, fans everywhere, and two small medical rooms.

J.W. was in the back room happily playing the air guitar while a couple of nurses checked his vital signs.

The doctor walked in and commanded, "Let me see his vitals."

He began to read them out loud, as if he was speaking to himself. "At 8:05 p.m., blood pressure 64/33, pulse 118. At 8:15 p.m. 68/37, pulse 116. At 8:25 p.m. 70/40, pulse 111."

It was now approaching 8:30 p.m. and the doctor wanted to take his own set of vital signs. "Somebody give me your blood pressure cuff and stethoscope." After taking the readings he announced, "Now he's 67/29 and pulse 114. How long has he been like this? We need to get him to Charity Hospital!"

Walking out of the room, the doctor tried to use his cell phone, which didn't work. Nearly all cell phone service in the New Orleans region had been knocked out by the storm. With the frustration mounting on his face, he blurted out, "Goddammit! I'll be back. I'm going to try and find Dr. Franks and Dr. Goddard and see if we can find a flat boat or something so we can get him to Charity!"

Meanwhile, I overheard some deputies talking about a ranking official in another building who had a heart attack, and many of the inmates were starting to riot. The situation continued to unravel.

"They're trying to burn down that mother fucker across the street," I heard a deputy telling another deputy.

"They got rank and deputies fallin' out over there!"

"This is getting fucked up around here!"

I went over to the narrow window to see if I could look down the street. It was pitch black, but catty-corner from our building, a fire burned brightly, lighting a tier on the third floor of one of the Templeman buildings.

A half -hour later, we'd received no word from the doctor. I could barely make out the water level outside the building, but I couldn't see my car or my dad's. I grabbed a flashlight from one of the deputies and shined it in the direction of our cars, hoping to see if they were flooded. They looked all right — so far. I went to find my dad and let him know the good news.

Making my way back to our spot, I found him listening to the radio with a deputy and her boyfriend. They had set up their stuff next to our spot.

"Done playing cards?"

"Yeah, I was getting tired."

"Are you feeling all right?"

"Yeah, just tired. ..."

"I'll get off of work in a couple of hours. Do you need anything?"

"You got any chocolate or candy?"

What is the deal with old people and sweets? Laughing a little, I said, "No, but I'll ask around and see if I can find you some. I'll see you later."

"I've got a Twix bar if you want it," a female deputy whispered to me.

She put it in my hand without my dad seeing her do it.

"Here you go, Dad!"

Befuddled, he asked, "How did you get one that fast?" It's always a little bit of fun to fool old folks and children.

"Magic, Dad. Magic!"

Turning back to the deputy, I whispered, "Thanks. I'll give you one back later."

With half a laugh and a smile, in a hushed voice she said,"Don't worry about it Gavin. We'll keep an eye on your dad."

"Thanks a lot," I softly replied. "Hey Dad, I'll be back in a couple of hours."

With his mouth half-full of the candy bar, he said, "Okay, Son. See you later."

Over by the second floor clinic, I saw the three doctors huddled together talking. I could only assume they were trying to decide what to do about our Elvis.

"Hey guys, what's up?" I asked.

"Well, we're working on getting a boat. We have a ranking officer and a deputy over at one of the other buildings who are both having medical problems, so we may have to bring all three in a boat to Charity."

"I hate to mention it, but we have another inmate on the 10th floor who got into a fight and has a cut above his left eye," I said.

"How bad is it?" one of the doctors asked. He had a demonstrative "here we go again" look on his face.

"I Steri-Stripped it and covered it. He could probably use three to five stitches." Steri-Strips are generally used to keep a laceration intact until a doctor can look at it and stitch it up. Or, if the cut is small enough, it can be used to help it close and heal.

"Oh, great. Somebody find Dr. Marcus and get him to go check the wound and do the stitches," Dr. Inglese said.

"I'll go find him and go up to 10. Y'all gonna take care of J.W.?" I asked.

"We've got it. Go ahead." With that, I started to ask around to see if anyone knew where Dr. Marcus was. I eventually found him and a nurse on the fourth floor treating an inmate who was having an asthma attack. I could barely see because it was so dark. The doctor was dealing with about as much as he could handle and I hated to say anything. "Hey, Doc. What's going on here?"

Looking very tired, he said, "We're treating this guy for asthma. We're about to take him to the second floor for a breathing treatment. What's going on with you?"

"We've got a guy on 10 who might need some stitches."

"When I'm done here I'll be up there. Give me a couple of minutes."

"All right. I'm heading up now."

The stairwell was hot and muggy, but the inmate chanting seemed to have quietened down. Making my way up the stairs, it hit me that I hadn't spoken to my wife since the previous afternoon. Lora and I had only been married a couple years, and when we were apart, we tried to talk to each other as much as possible. With the situation rapidly deteriorating, I was desperate to talk with her.

The 10th floor phone system was still working at that point, and I hurried up the stairs to call her cell phone. Of course, the call didn't go through. I grabbed my wallet to look for the number of the hotel in Tyler, Texas, where she was staying. After a couple busy signals, the call finally went through, and I got the hotel operator.

"I need room 107, I think."

"Hold, please."

After a half-dozen rings there was no answer, so I hung up.

As I was looking for Debbie's (my sister-in-law) number, my cell phone surprisingly rang. It was Lora, thank goodness. "Hey, babe. Is everything all right?" she asked.

Still catching my breath from climbing up the stairs I replied, "Well, I'm alive. It's been crazy around here. The inmates are shaking the bars, chanting, fighting and getting rowdy. We've got a guy who might be dying; there's water everywhere on the 10th floor; I heard a deputy might have had a heart attack; a nurse had an asthma attack; we got ..."

"Hey, hey, slow down a minute. Are you okay, Gavin?"

Breathing deeply, I said, "Yeah, I'm ... good ... ah ... just a little out of breath."

"Why?"

"Well, the elevators aren't working, so I have ... to go up and down the ... stairs from ten to two and other floors in between... between all the madness and checking on my dad. I'm getting tired of running these stairs."

"You better slow down. I don't want anything to happen to you."

"I'll be all right. Hey listen, the phones are probably going to go out, so if I can't get through to you, that's the reason."

After an extended silence, Lora said, "I love you baby ... be ... safe. ..."

I could hear her voice cracking a little, which gave me a lump in my throat. "I'll be all right. Take care. Kiss the dogs, say 'hi' to everyone for me, and don't worry. I think the storm has passed. Oh yeah, I almost forgot, it looks like our cars avoided the flood waters. There's about three to four feet of water surrounding our buildings, but our cars are in the highest spot in the parking lot."

With some hesitation in her voice, she said, "Th ... that's great. Hopefully, you'll be able ... to ... leave ... soon." I could tell she was beginning to cry.

"Are you crying? Please don't ... I'll be fine, " I reassured her.

"What ...about your dad?"

"So far, he's all right. I think he now realizes he should have left. The only bad thing is he's running out of medicine."

"Hopefully, y'all won't be there too long."

I tried to be strong. "That would be nice. I'm just wondering how long it's gonna take for this water to go down. Anyway, I better get going. I love you. Take care and I'll talk to you soon."

"Bye, baby ... I love you ... so much. Miss you."

"Love you. Miss you too. Bye-bye." Hanging up the phone, I could hear the female inmates had started yelling again.

The deputies appeared to be nowhere in sight. Walking over there and trying not to slip and fall with all the water on the floor, I heard someone say, "Who's there?"

Startled, I answered, "It's Nurse Johnson. Who's that?"

"Dr. Singh," the feminine voice replied with her foreign accent.

"Oh, hey, Dr. Singh. I heard these crazy women screaming and hollering over there and I came to see what was going on with them."

Dr. Singh is one of our psychiatrists and she was on the 10th floor, sleeping on a cot in the back office. "Hello Nurse Johnson. I was just taking a nap in the back, and I heard the screaming also. What's going on?"

"I have no idea. I don't see any deputies anywhere. I'm gonna go down the tier and see what the problem is."

As nurses, we're not supposed to open any of the security gates. Since there were no deputies around, and there was someone screaming, I took it upon myself to open the gate to see what the problem was.

"What's wrong? Who's screaming down there?"

A female voice yelled, "The girl in my cell is having a seizure or somethin'!"

After popping the gate open, I carefully ran down the slippery hallway to see a twitching and unconscious female on the cell floor. She was unresponsive to my questions.

"How long has she been like this?"

"Man, I don't know. Five minutes maybe or somethin' like that."

I opened the cell, which I obviously wasn't supposed to do, but I had no choice. I entered with Dr. Singh looking over my shoulder.

I said, "All right, I'm gonna roll her on her side. I'm going to need you to keep her on her side while I go get some help, all right?"

With some hesitation, the inmate replied, "Yeah, yeah, all right, man!"

Rushing to the medical office, I got a wheelchair and some ammonia capsules (sometimes called smelling salts), which are used to help someone wake up, and we often use them to see if an inmate is faking a seizure as they sometimes do — imagine that! If someone is faking it, which happens quite a bit in the incarcerated environment, the person will react as if bleach or something like that was stuck up his or her nose. People having real seizures will be unresponsive or slow to respond, and their eyes may roll back in their heads. They may also urinate or defecate on themselves.

By the time I got back she was somewhat responsive, and after I put the ammonia capsule under her nose she started to speak.

"What the fuck? SHIT! What the hell is that shit, man?!"

I asked, "You feelin' all right? Stay still and let me get some vital signs on you."

Her blood pressure was 134/85 and her pulse was 110. Respirations were 18 per minute (borderline elevated)and her temperature was 99. Based on the vital signs, which were pretty normal, she may or may not have had a seizure. I began asking her a series of questions that could help me determine whether she was being honest or not.

"Do you have seizure disorder?"

"Yeah, I have 'caesars,'" she pronounced it.

"What do you take for your seizures?"

"I take them Dilantin 100s and Phenobarbital 30s," she replied, referring to the dosages.

"When was the last time you took your meds?"

"Well, I just got arrested two days ago and these bitches around here won't give me my meds. I guess I took them about a week ago."

"A week ago? If you've only been in jail for two days and your last meds were a week ago, what happened to the five days in between?"

"Well, you know ... I don't know man ... I was partying before I came to jail."

"Were you doing any drugs before you came to jail?"

A devilish smile came over her face and she looked me straight in the eye and said, "No sir! Not me!"

Obviously, I couldn't believe that part of her story, so I countered, "Yeah, right. So if we did a drug test it would show up negative, right?"

"Why you givin' me a hard time now, man? You gonna help me or what?"

"Yes. Get in this wheelchair so I can bring you to the office."

One of the requirements of the medical field is that everything that happens to patients or, in this case, inmates, has to be documented. We have to write nurses' notes, usually with vital signs and the time and date the incidents occur, along with detailed descriptions of what happened. In hospitals, this is essential because people are in the hospital because they are sick. In a correctional facility, inmates usually are not sick initially, but when something happens, a nurse is still expected to document it. Workers in the medical field are always open to lawsuits, and if things are not documented, a lawyer can use that against us. Most occurrences in a corrections setting are not life-threatening, but the area I work in — psychiatry — is unique. People often try to kill themselves when they are in jail, so we take every threat seriously. If someone wants to take his or her own life, we don't want it to happen in jail. We have to protect those people from themselves as well as others.

Everything that happened earlier with J.W. and the other medical incidents had to be documented. We take every incident as if it were a true medical crisis. I brought the woman to the medical office, and Dr. Marcus and a nurse walked in at the same time. "Where's the guy with the laceration?" the doctor inquired.

Trying to compose myself a bit, I said, "Give me a minute, Doc. I have this female inmate here who may have had a seizure. She said she takes Dilantin and Phenobarbital, but hasn't taken her medication in a week. Can I get an order for both?"

Looking fatigued, he said, "Yeah. Get me her chart, and I'll write an order. In the meantime, give her a loading dose of 400 mg of Dilantin now, another 300 mg in four hours, and another 200 mg in another four hours."

"Okay, Doc. Thanks."

The inmate was stable enough to walk, so I gave her the medication and got one more set of vital signs — for documentation purposes — and walked her back to her cell. I was now playing nurse and deputy. After locking her cell, it seemed like every female all of a sudden had a problem.

"Come here, white boy!"

"My head hurts! Damn!"

"I'm in pain! You gotta help me!"

Walking off the tier, I had to ignore all the yelling and screaming about headaches and back pain and other feigned maladies. I called down to the Watch Commander's office. After a few rings, someone picked up the phone and with some frustration in my voice, I asked, "Will y'all send a deputy or somebody up to 10? The doctor is up here, and we have somebody who needs stitches."

"Who the hell is this?" grumbled the unfamiliar voice.

"Nurse Gavin. There's no deputy up here and we need one ASAP!"

"No deputy? Hang on. We'll have one up there in a minute."

I knew this would take a while because the elevators were out. There aren't too many deputies who will feel like walking up eight flights of stairs in the heat.

"Hey, Dr. M., you ever see so much stuff goin' on at one time?" I asked.

Looking at me and half-heartedly smiling, he said, "No, I can't say I have. This is pretty wild!"

Deciding to make small talk, I offered, "Did you hear about the Twin Spans? I heard they're totally destroyed."

"What? You kidding?" The smile melted from his face.

Pointing to the radio in the other office, I said, "That's what WWL (local station 870 AM, our news source during and after the storm) said."

Immediately following the hurricane and for weeks afterward, most of the city's radio stations combined their resources and personnel into a single 24-hour broadcast on multiple frequencies, both AM and FM. We only got one reporting source, and the facts and details were often confusing. Sometimes, we heard gut-wrenching, heart-breaking pleas for help from stranded residents.

"That's unbelievable," the doctor replied. "I wonder if the other roadways are damaged too."

"I don't know, I only heard about the Twin Spans." "Where's this guy with the laceration above his eye?"

"I had to call downstairs to get Rank to send up a deputy. We're security-free up here."

"Oh, that's just great." Dr. Marcus then stood up and looked around for a second or two and asked, "Is there an outside phone line that works up here?"

"Yeah. Try that phone in the office over there."

"I'll be right back."

Meanwhile, I saw Nurse Favis on her cell phone in the corner of the soaked office, looking out the window as she spoke.

"Hey Favis, you can go back downstairs if you want. I got it up here," I said.

"You sure?"

"Yeah. When you go down, pass by the Watch Office and tell them the doctor is up here and we need a deputy up here, please."

"No problem. See you later."

It was about 10:45 p.m., and it was starting to calm down a little bit inside the prison. I could hear a few arguments and inmates being loud, but that was common on the 10th floor. Normally, I could close the door and turn on the air conditioning. Since the air conditioner was now sitting on the floor, that wasn't an option. With no a/c, and all the moisture and puddles on the floor, this office was the last place I wanted to be. Taking a walk around to the south side of the 10th floor, I looked out of one of the small windows.

It was so dark inside it looked like I was in a closed closet with the light off. It was spooky to see nothing but darkness outside and various buildings on fire. The fires were scattered all over as far as I could see. I could barely see a small part of what appeared to be the moon. Faint traces of clouds floated by, but no rain. At that moment, a part of me couldn't wait for the morning to get a real look at the city.

The House of Detention building I was in is 10 stories high. The view includes parts of the Central Business District downtown, Uptown, and Mid-City during the daylight hours. I was feeling pretty confident our cars were still all right. Some of the employees parked on the street and the employee lot was full. The problem was the street and the front part of the employee lot are quite low. Most of New Orleans is below sea level, and elevations are often spoken of in inches, rather than feet. Inches can make a difference when a heavy downpour floods the streets. I was sure those cars in the employee lot would be flooded or have at least a little water in them. The employee lot is a big one that holds 300 to 400 cars and has a pretty good slope to it. As I mentioned, we had parked in the highest possible spot, so if ours got flooded then all the other cars would already be under water.

I was mesmerized by a blazing fire that appeared to be near St. Charles Avenue, a majestic boulevard from Downtown to Uptown New Orleans, running past Tulane and Loyola universities. Referred to by locals as simply, "the avenue," St. Charles is beautifully lined with dancing live oak trees and magnificent mansions, with streetcars rolling through the middle.

I heard footsteps coming up the stairs. The deputy had finally arrived. We could get those stitches done, and I could go back downstairs to get some sleep.

Breathlessly, the deputy said, "Y'all … got... someone ... who's ... cut. Damn, that's a long-ass haul up those steps!"

"Tell me about it. I've been walkin' those steps all day," I answered. "Do me a favor, go get H.B. on the south side, cell seven for me, please."

"Where do you want him?" he panted.

Pointing to my right, I said, "On the bench, right there.

The doc is going to stitch him up real quick."

"All right. You got it, G."

Dr. Marcus was still on the phone, but he wasn't speaking. I waited for a minute or so before I said anything. "Doc, we've got the inmate ready for the stitches."

"All right, give me a minute." The inmate was cooperating, thank God, so I was able to remove the bandage easily to see how the cut looked. Dr. Marcus hung up the phone and took four or five steps toward us before slipping forward directly into the medicine cart was near us. Fortunately, he caught himself before he fell in the puddle of water that caused him to slip in the first place.

"Goddammit! What the hell? That would have capped my day off just right."

"Don't feel bad; I slipped at least two or three times today. This is an accident waiting to happen," I said.

The inmate with the laceration was also one of our regulars. He's a paranoid schizophrenic who is constantly getting into fights with other inmates, having a knack for hurting the hands of the inmates with his face. Surprisingly, he was calm at the time, so I hoped things would go smoothly.

"Gavin, please get me a small laceration kit, a number 4.0 Vicryl stitch, Lidocaine, and a five-eighth length needle," Dr. Marcus said.

"I'll be right back," I said, taking a mental note of his request.

Our medical supply room is very small on the 10th floor and not well stocked. After looking for a few minutes, I realized we only had laceration kits and no stitches of any kind.

Exhausted and agitated, I said, "Hey Doc, I'm gonna have to go to the second floor clinic to get some stitches. I'll be back." Walking down the stairs, I tried to figure out how many times I'd been up and down them that day. All I knew was that I'd sleep well that night.

Chapter 10

Aftermath

The second-floor clinic was getting noisier and noisier, filling up with employees' families who were moving out of the cafeteria area. There were some volatile people in there, and patience was running short. After navigating my way around the sleeping bags and mattresses on the floor, I was able to get to the medical supply room. A family was set up in there, blocking the cabinet where the stitches were kept. There were two small children sleeping, so I tip-toed around them and grabbed the box of stitches.

By this point, I was thirsty and hungry. Nurse Favis was eating a sandwich — which looked awfully good.

"Whatcha' eatin'?" I asked.

"Hot sausage sandwich. You want one?"

"Hell, yeah. You don't mind?"

"Gavin, you know you're my boy. I just got to cook it up right quick."

Right near the front of the clinic was a refrigerator and a portable electric burner with a frying pan on top.

"Don't worry about it. I didn't know you had to cook it."

"That's all right, G; it'll only take a couple of minutes. What do you want on it? We got mayo, mustard, lettuce, and tomatoes."

"Everything but tomatoes."

"Comin' right up!"

The loud sizzling and smell of sausage frying filled the room. I could hear people talking in the main corridor about the different things they were hearing on the radio about The Storm and its aftermath.

"You got somethin' to drink?" Favis asked.

"Nope; let me go over by my stuff. I have some water over there. I'll be right back," I said.

"I'll have your sandwich ready when you get back."

The hallway was dimly lit, since we were running off of a diesel-powered generator and only a few lights were on to conserve energy.

My dad was asleep and Deputy Jeanne's boyfriend was lying across from him, listening to the radio. Grabbing my blue duffel bag and opening it up, I whispered to him, "I just came to get some water."

"That's cool. You been runnin' around all day, huh?" he asked.

Shaking my head and raising my eyebrows, I replied, "You have no idea. It's been crazy around here today. Thank God it's almost over. I'll be back in a little while."

"Later G..."

After gobbling up the hot sausage sandwich, I made my way up the stairs once again. This time I brought a flashlight just in case.

When I got back to the 10th floor, I could hear someone hollering.

When is this crap gonna end?

Turning the corner, I saw a deputy holding the inmate who needed stitches face down on the floor with the doctor standing over him chuckling a little bit.

"What's wrong with this idiot?" I asked.

The deputy turned to me and said, "All of the sudden he started freakin' out and yelling, 'Don't kill me, Don't kill me.'

Then he lunged at the doc."

Dr. Marcus smiled and nodded.

"Well, Doc, do you want to do these stitches or what?"

Darting his eye at me, he said, "Let him calm down a minute."

Before he could finish what he was saying, the disturbed inmate started yelling, "Help me! Help me! Don't kill me! Please!" This went on for a few minutes. Finally, I was able to convince the inmate we were trying to help him.

"All right, let's get this over with," Dr. Marcus said. As he set up the Lidocaine to deaden the cut, the inmate went berserk. "No, no! Stop, Please!"

At this point, Dr. Marcus shouted, "Fuck it! Get a medical refusal form and let's sign it! He is obviously not going to let me do anything! You can Steri-Strip the cut when he calms down. He's all right."

After we both signed the form and had the deputy sign it as a witness, I put it in his chart.

The doctor said he was leaving. "See ya later Dr. Marcus." I said apologetically.

"Bye."

The situation was wearing on him.

The inmate sat on the bench, rocking back and forth while staring at the floor. Mumbling to himself, he appeared to be calming down.

"Harold, I'm going to cover your cut up, okay?" At first he didn't answer. I waited a second or two and tried again. "Hey Harold, look up for me please!" He looked up. The deputy handcuffed him and sat him straight up.

Harold then very calmly said, "You may do as you please." His change in demeanor was a little freaky, but I Steri-Stripped his cut and covered it with a bandage. After I was finished, the deputy put Harold back in his cell.

Nurse Donna came through the door by the stairwell. She was obviously out of breath and sat down in the medical office.

"Damn, that's a hot-ass stairwell! It took me 15 minutes to get up those damn stairs," she said, trying to catch her breath.

I smiled, "You want me to call the doctor? I can give you a breathing treatment if you need it."

Laughing back at me, she said, "Kiss my big black ass!"

I gave her a rundown of the evening's events, and she told me about some things she had heard on the radio. After leaving the 10th floor and walking the stairs for that last time that night, I thought about Lora and our puppies. Then it hit me that I also hadn't spoken to my mother in several days.

My mom works for Amtrak, and I didn't know if she had evacuated or not. She doesn't have a cell phone, so I couldn't call her. I thought I remembered her saying she was leaving over the weekend (before the hurricane) for Chicago on the City of New Orleans train.

My mother Roberta had come to New Orleans from Chicago for Mardi Gras when she was 19. She met my dad, at the time a jazz musician at the Blue Room. He was nearly 30 years her senior. He helped her through some difficult situations with a roommate and eventually they developed a relationship. Although they divorced when I was eight, my parents are still friends to this day.

My mom has another son, my younger half-brother Alex who is 19 and lives in the nearby coastal town of Waveland, Mississippi. I don't get to see him very often because he lives with his father, and I hadn't talked to him in a while. I said a little prayer and hoped he was all right too. Many people were in my situation. Calls couldn't go in or out for the most part. The uncertainty was agonizing.

My family was on my mind as I walked the stairs with my flashlight on. Before I knew it, I had walked too far and found myself confused and standing in a stairwell just above the first floor level.

I pointed my flashlight down right below my feet and could see water, about a foot or so, just above the first step. Making my way back up to the second floor, I saw a female deputy walking with a towel around her head and a bottle of shampoo in her hand. Her "at home" presence was a stark contrast to the conditions. As she turned the corner I asked, "Where can we take a shower?"

She acted like she didn't hear me because she kept walking.

Was I seeing things?

I saw Deputy Henry by the side door to the Watch Office. "Hey Henry, can we take a shower somewhere?"

Looking both ways before saying anything, he whispered, "Get your stuff, come back here and you can take a shower."

Our things were not far away and as I approached the disorganized pile I was sure to be as quiet as I could so I didn't wake my dad. My bags were at the end of my air mattress, and Dad's foot was touching the edge of one of them. Thankfully, he was sound asleep and snoring. I grabbed my towel, a change of clothes, and my shampoo. Deputy Henry was by the side door when I got back, and he opened it quickly, telling me to hurry up. Obviously, the shower was for the deputies only, not the medical staff.

"Thanks a lot. I'm dying for a shower," I said.

"Hey G, the only problem is there's no hot water."

"That's all right, I've been sweating all day; I could use it."

The shower stall was tiny with a very small, drippy shower head. It was smelly, dark, and dingy. I turned on the water, and, surprisingly it came out in a fairly strong stream. The deputy wasn't kidding, the water was ice cold! I put my flip-flops on and stepped into the shower. "Ooh, ooh! Damn that's cold!" It was like somebody pouring a pitcher of ice water on my head. I jumped out and stood there naked with tensed muscles and my head nearly frozen, then eased my way back into the shower. I quickly soaped up and shampooed my head, but it didn't lather well.

After the showering in record time, I got dressed and made my way back to my "comfy" air mattress. My dad was still sleeping soundly, and it was fairly quiet. I checked my cellphone one more time, and it read 12:05 a.m. Thinking we might be stranded a little while, I shut it off to conserve the battery and rolled over to try and sleep.

I could hear the sounds of assorted radios with newscasters talking about the aftermath of the storm. I listened to the grim reality of the surrounding area. Apparently, the storm took a slight turn to the east and the Gulfport-Biloxi, Mississippi area, about 60 miles east of New Orleans, took a direct hit. They had 30-foot storm surges from the Gulf that washed away entire blocks of waterfront houses.

That also meant Waveland had been hit hard – where my brother lives. He doesn't live far from the beach, so all I could hope for was that he evacuated. I knew my mother would be very worried about him.

The announcer on the radio sounded very grim, "... the Twin Span bridges are gone ... destroyed ... the city of Slidell, Louisiana ... inundated with water ... massive devastation! We have word that the Gulf Coast region of Mississippi is obliterated. Gone. Some estimates have the storm surge as high as 50 feet ... We have reports that some of the levees in New Orleans have given way ... the pumps have failed ... there are dead bodies floating in the streets of the city ... dogs running wild ... People are calling from their attics pleading for help ..."

I listened for a half-hour or so. With each passing moment, the sinking feeling in my stomach got deeper and deeper. It looked like we were stuck. Taking one last look at my dad before I tried to get some sleep, I rolled over again and said another little prayer.

What's next?

Chapter 11

Surroundings

I woke in the darkness around 5 a.m. to my dad rummaging through his duffel bag. It felt like I had just laid my head down to sleep.

Whatcha' lookin' for, Dad?"

"My medicine. I can't see real good … You got a flashlight?"

Lying on the other side of us was Nurse Urban and his mother. This lady was a piece of work. I would come to appreciate the things she would do as the time went by. Urban said, "Mr. Johnson, I have a flashlight for you. Here you go."

"Oh, thank you." My dad leaned over and whispered close to my left ear, "I gotta' take a dump!"

Realizing it would be dark in the bathroom, I told him I would go with him. It was only about 25 feet from where we were set up. Everybody in our section of the building used this bathroom and, up until this point, it still worked.

Whispering, I said, "Dad, give me the flashlight, put your hand on my shoulder and follow me.

Once we got to the bathroom, we saw that it was pretty dark and starting to smell like a foul public toilet.

"Dad, make sure you clean the seat before you sit."

"Yeah, I got it."

I could hear him straining a little. "I think I'm constipated Son. I don't have my Sun-Chlorella pills – I forgot them when I was packing. They help me go to the bathroom and keep me young." In the past, he had told me about those pills.

He swears they make him look and feel younger.

"I thought those were the pills that make you look younger; I didn't know they were a laxative too."

"Everybody I meet can't believe that I'm 83 — they think I'm 50 to 55 years old!"

"Come on Dad, 50 years old?"

"I'm telling you Son. These pills do all kinds of things for me."

After a couple more unpleasant, but funny, sounds, he said, "Y'all got anything to help me go?"

Trying not to laugh, I said, "We should. Do you want me to look now?"

"No. Later." With that, he buckled up and we went back to bed. After fumbling around in the dark, I said, "Wait here and I'll be right back."

The second-floor clinic was dark and very quiet. There were people lying just about everywhere on the floor. The medicine carts were in the back, of course, so I once again tiptoed around everyone on the floor. The carts were full of just about everything a medical staff person could need. People who are incarcerated often get better medical treatment than they would get if they weren't in jail.

One of the nurses heard me. "Who's there? What are you looking for?"

"It's Gavin. My dad needs a laxative."

"Look in the bottom right-hand drawer. There's some magnesium citrate. That'll help him." Procedures were out the window at this point. We were keeping the medicine secure from having a free-for-all, but survival was the name of the game. My dad's health was definitely priority.

"Thanks."

I decided to go to the break room to see the water level outside the building. The visibility was poor, but I could see the rising waters were getting closer to our cars. Some cars were already almost completely covered, but ours were still safe. How deep could this get?

It was daybreak and looking like it was going to be a nice day. The sun was just starting to shine and, amazingly, there were no clouds. Walking back over by my dad, I noticed there were a few people moving around, but for the most part, everyone was still asleep. I walked over by the front entrance and saw Nurse Cecilia and her family talking.

"Hey Gavin, what's going on?"

"Nothing much. Looks like we survived another storm."

"I guess so ..."

In her Southern drawl she asked, "How's your daddy?"

"He seems to be okay. I'm sure he wishes he would haveevacuated."

In unison, four members of her family and Cecilia all said, "Us too!"

After some laughter, Cecilia asked, "You heard about them levees?"

"I heard something on the radio about them failing orsomething. Why? What did you hear?" I asked.

"Oh yeah, I heard over by Lake Pontchartrain and also Chalmette (a suburb of New Orleans to the southeast of the city where Cecilia lives) was fillin' up with water."

"You heard anything about Kenner?" I was worried about my home.

"Not yet, but if I do I'll let you know ... if you're hungry, I heard they're makin' some breakfast over by the kitchen."

"All right, thanks. See you later."

It was about 6:30 a.m. or so, and I left to see if they really were making breakfast. It sure sounded good. The break room was starting to get a few stragglers, and just about everyone was taking turns looking out of the window. It seemed everyone, like me, wanted to see if cars were flooded or not.

"Aw, Jesus, man. My car is gone!" someone yelled out.

"Don't feel bad — mine too," another voice echoed from the back of the room. The consensus seemed to be that everyone's car had taken some water.

Patiently waiting my turn, I saw the water was touching my dad's car tire, about a quarter of the way up. Mine was parked right next to his with the water barely touching my tire. I was feeling pretty good that our cars were safe, since the storm was gone and the skies looked like they would be clear for the day. Looking to my right, I could see about three or four cars with the back windows blown out or shattered. I overheard someone say they saw the wind blow parts of the exhaust vents off the Templeman buildings, a couple of the main buildings within the local penal system, that landed on those cars, smashing out some of the back windows. Since those cars were in the back of the parking lot, they had survived the initial flooding, but not the flying vents. The parking lot was beginning to look like a big dirty swimming pool, with hundreds of flooded cars in it. Some of the cars had started to float about.

It was about this time one of the ranking officials came in and said, "Breakfast will be served between 7:30 and eight in the old cafeteria area." Some people immediately left to get in line while others rushed to notify their families breakfast was about to be served. Instead of rushing, I took my time to get my dad. I figured I'd let him sleep a little longer.

It was close to eight o'clock. I was reading one of my books while lying on my mattress when my father woke up. "Hey Dad, you want some breakfast?"

"Yeah, what do they have?"

"I don't know. We have to grab a plate over near the old cafeteria and get in line. Come on, it'll be like Piccadilly's." Piccadilly's is a Southern cafeteria chain my father lists as one of his favorites.

Looking a little confused he said, "Hold on a second, let me put on my shoes."

The line was long and filled with all kinds of characters — young, old, big, small, black, white, yellow, and everything in between. During the night, they must have hung a tarp to separate the cafeteria from the kitchen. Looking at some of the passersby, I could see they were serving runny oatmeal, a bright red hot dog, and a hard-boiled egg. It was readily apparent this was not going to be a very tasty breakfast. “Well, Dad, this won’t be McDonald’s, but it’ll have to do.”

“That’s all right, Son. I’m hungry.”

The line slowly moved along and after 10 minutes or so, we got our food and went down the hallway to eat.

“How is it, Dad?”

“Not bad.”

“You want my oatmeal? I’m not a big oatmeal eater.”

“Sure, put it here,” he said, pointing to an empty spot on his plate. As I slid the runny oatmeal off my plate, I saw others doing the same. The oatmeal didn’t seem to be popular with the young people.

After breakfast, I gave my dad a few swigs of the magnesium citrate. “This should do the trick. Give it a couple of hours to work, all right?”

He nodded and said, “Where’s the front door?” reaching in his pocket for a cigarette.

“Why? Do you want to smoke?”

“Well ... um ... I just want to get some fresh air.”

I played along.

I had seen a few people the day before smoking by the front entrance to the building, but it was now under two feet of water.

“Wait here and I’ll go find out.”

I went to the Watch Commander’s office. I was instructed to go by the inmate visitors’ center, which is near the front entrance on the second floor. I went to go back and get my dad, but he was gone. "Has anybody seen my dad?"

A couple of people pointed toward the second-floor clinic. I went over there, but he wasn't there. I was walking toward the break room when I saw him coming out of the unisex bathroom. Agitated by now, I said, "I told you to wait and I'd be right back. You didn't smoke in that bathroom did you?" "Yeah. Why? What's the big deal?"

"You're not at home. You can't just do whatever you want in here. This is a jail and if somebody sees you doing that then everybody will start doing what he or she wants, and we can't have that here. Come follow me, and I'll show you where to go next time." It's funny; for the last few years my dad has felt the need to try to hide the fact he smokes. He's been smoking for 50-plus years and had a mild stroke in 1998. When I go to visit him on my off days, he sometimes is smoking when I look through the window before I come in. When I come through the door, he cups the cigarette in his hand and plays dumb like a teenager, while smoke is coming from under his hand. Or he'll hear the door opening and get up and walk to the back of the house so I can't see him. I know what he's doing, but I go along with him. He knows I don't smoke, and I don't approve of him smoking, but I would never tell him what to do. I mean, he's made it to his 80s, right? I have to give him credit though; he has slacked off a bit, and he's definitely more aware of his health.

The environment we were in was bad enough, so I couldn't really blame him for wanting a cigarette, and I could tell he was uncomfortable. I had tried to tell him what it was going to be like at the jail. If it was just me, it wouldn't be so bad, but having to keep track of him was stressing me out and creating tension between us. I didn't like treating him like a child, but I felt I needed to keep an eye on him.

"I'm gonna go up to the 10th floor to see how things are going." Jokingly, I added, "Stay out of trouble." He smiled and started to walk down to the visitors' area.

I told myself I would keep count of how many times I went up and down the stairs that day. Hopefully, it wouldn't be like the day before. Walking up the stairs, I took a look down from the second floor to the ground floor, and I could see that the water level was about halfway up the first set of stairs. I thought that was a little strange since the storm was long gone. The water should have been receding, not rising. What I didn't know was that because of the levee breaks by Lake Pontchartrain, the entire city was filling up with millions of gallons of water ... contaminated with oil, gas, sewage and rotting corpses.

The stairwell was really hot for so early in the morning, and I was going to make every effort to not make that hike if I could avoid it. The 10th floor was fairly calm when I got up there. I had forgotten we had taken in some St. Bernard Parish (a suburb adjacent to New Orleans) inmates and their deputies. They were housed on the 10th floor in the holding cell, an area about 20 by 25 feet. There were five or six deputies in there.

After observing the cramped situation, I decided to introduce myself. "Hey guys (there were actually a couple of females also), I'm Gavin, and I'm one of the nurses up here." They all introduced themselves and gave me a rundown of who was who and what they were there for.

"Make yourselves comfortable and if there's anything I can do, just let me know." A couple of nurses were in the waterlogged medical office, trying to clean up a little.

"What's up, y'all?" I asked.

In unison, they said, "Help!"

"Hold on just a minute," I replied.

Before I got started, I decided to try and call Lora. My cell phone had no signal, so I used the office phone. As you might imagine, the landline was dead too. I realized it would be a while before I would speak to her again. I was really missing her. A lot.

I regretted going up there because for the next couple of hours, I was mopping up water and moving things around. After helping to clean up, I went back to the second floor to check on my dad. It was about 11 a.m., and it was getting hotter by the minute. There were two big fans set up in the middle corridor that circulated the hot, humid air, and the door was open in an attempt to cool the building.

Looking through the door, I could see water and what looked like raw sewage backing up through the drains in the recreation area outside. On a positive note, opening the door to the stairwell and having the fans on was helping with the air circulation and helped cool off the building somewhat. But they were also blowing the foul smells about.

My dad was near our area reading the newspaper from the weekend before the storm. I asked him if he was hungry, but he said he wasn't. With the stench around us, I wasn't really hungry either.

I decided to find somebody with a radio and ventured over to the right side of our area. I introduced myself to a young African-American man and his pregnant wife. "Hey, how are you doing? My name's Gavin. Do you mind if I listen to the radio with you?"

"Hey man, I'm T.C. and this is my wife. Have a seat," he said. We got to talking, and I was quickly impressed with him.

He said he just graduated from Loyola Law School, recently took the bar exam, and was headed into the Air Force as a lawyer. "I'm waiting to get my bar exam results, and then we're moving to Virginia."

I asked, "How do you think you did?"

"Oh, I feel pretty good about it man. I'm pretty confident I passed it. It was a bitch though."

"I bet. Now, how did you end up here?"

"My mom is Mrs. Chaisson. She works in the Watch Office."

It took me a second to realize who he was talking about, but then it hit me, "Oh, yeah, I know her."

The radio announcer started talking about the levee breaks. "We have confirmation that there is a levee break at the Seventeenth Street Canal in Lakeview (an affluent area of New Orleans near Lake Pontchartrain) ...also, levee breaks at the Industrial Canal in the lower Ninth Ward (a poor area of New Orleans) ... There is a failure at the London Street Canal and Chalmette is under 10 to 20 feet of water. I repeat, we have levee failures at ..."

Sitting down on the old, dirty floor I didn't know what to think. After a few seconds of reflection, I felt like I myself was in prison. We weren't going anywhere.

T.C. got up and paced around a little bit. "This is some bullshit, man."

"You ain't lying. I'll be right back. I'm gonna go tell my dad the bad news."

I went back over to where my dad was. Looking out the window at the water surrounding our building, I said, "Hey dad, it looks like we're going to be here a while."

A little confused, he asked, "We're not going home later? The storm is over isn't it?"

"Yeah the storm's over, but the levees have broken all over town. Water is pouring into the city."

"We're not close to any levees. We'll be able to leave later ..."

"Have you looked out the window lately? We're surrounded by water. We're not going anywhere!"

With a disturbed look, he asked, "How are our cars?"

"Come take a walk with me and I'll show you. When I checked earlier they were all right."

I thought about walking him up to the 10th floor so he could get a look at the flooded city with fires burning and all that stuff, but I figured I'd spare him. We went to the break room instead. It was packed with people playing cards and dominoes, and eating lunch.

"Come over here and look out this window — can you see your car?" I pointed in the direction of our cars.

"Damn. That water is pretty high. Is that my car over there?"

Pointing to the left I said, "One to the left in the back corner. See mine, the blue one?"

After a pause he said, "Oh yeah, it's okay. We'll be all right."

Incredulous, I said, "It's halfway up over your tires. See?"

"I can't see that far, Son. If it floods, it floods. What the hell?"

"I guess it depends on where the water flows. We'll have to wait and see."

Deciding to change the subject I asked him if he was hungry yet.

Looking at me somewhat apologetically, he said, "I could eat something, I guess."

Walking down the middle corridor, my dad stopped in front of the huge fan to cool off for a minute. It was nearing noontime, and the heat was stifling. Absolutely stifling. I worried about him. Once we got to "our area" I took my food bag and dumped it onto his mattress so he could pick something out to eat. He said he'd forgotten to go to the store (which I figured). I had a little extra food for both of us just in case. "I've got a couple cans of Hormel tamales here, two cans of soup, a can of raviolis, some pork and beans."

After touching everything I put on the mattress, he finally grabbed a can and said, "I'll eat so me tamales. They're not the spicy kind, are they? I can't eat anything too spicy."

"Nope. They're the regular kind. I'm going to put them in this Tupperware dish right here and go warm them up for you in the microwave."

Before I could finish, he said, "I need something to drink."

"I've got some lemonade or ice tea packs you can mix in a bottle of water."

"I'll take a tea. You got ice?"

"Yeah right dad! Look in that blue bag right there and grab a bottle of water."

I tried to fit as much water in my bag as I could, just in case. I brought two duffel bags and one small cooler bag filled with granola bars, drink packs, and canned food. Lora had insisted on it. I had clothes, water, and my portable DVD player with movies in it. Picking up the can of tamales and the can opener, I told my dad, "I'll be right back."

When I got to the break room, I saw that the microwave was gone. I asked one of the deputies where it was and he said, "They came and got it because it wasn't working."

I hastily replied, "I saw someone using it at breakfast." The deputy just shrugged his shoulders and left the break room. I went back by dad and told him the microwave was broken.

Not looking fazed, he said, "That's all right, son, I'll just eat 'em cold. I eat stuff cold a lot. It's not a big deal."

"You sure? I can try and find you a sandwich or something."

At that point, he reached up and took the dish right out of my hand, almost spilling it on him. He peeled the paper covering off each of the tamales, eating them with his fingers.

I was a little surprised by this and said, "Hold on a minute. I have a fork in my bag — here!" With his mouth half full and red juice on his finger and thumb, he took the fork and continued eating.

I chuckled a little to myself.

When he was finished he had one left and proceeded to wrap it in some sort of paper and save it for later. Old people with their "save anything" mentality! When he did this, it reminded me of a day about a year or so earlier when I was eating lunch at the golf course. My friend and I had just finished playing golf and had started to eat lunch when my dad walked into the clubhouse and sat down with us.

Corey had just finished eating a burger and had about 10 French fries left on his plate. Without even asking, my dad reached over and took a couple of fries off of his plate and proceeded to eat them. As he was chewing them he said to Corey, "You finished with those fries?"

With a big grin, Corey said, "I guess I am now! Why you want the rest?"

"Yeah, I think I'll take them home and eat them later."

Corey and I couldn't believe our eyes when my dad took to a napkin and put the few fries in it, roll it up and put it in his pocket.

Here's a guy who could go eat anywhere or better yet, order some food, but he decides to take a few French fries home for later. I tell you, old folks can really make you laugh. I guess his thriftiness was left over from surviving the Great Depression.

"You gonna eat that tamale later?"

"Oh, yeah, Son. Never waste food!"

Jokingly, I told him, "Save me a piece for later, all right?"

He looked at me a little funny, "You want a piece later?" "I'm just kidding with you, Pops — it's all yours." After that little bit of entertainment, I went back over by T.C. and the radio.

"Any other news?"

"You shoulda' heard what they were saying about the Superdome! They said some of the people over there are committing suicide; people are gettin' raped, killed! Complete chaos!" "What? You're kidding!" I was stunned. "They also said that part of the roof blew off the 'dome as well."

I was starting to get a bad mental picture of what the city looked like. It was falling apart, and there was no help on the way that I knew of. *Another silent prayer.*

For the next couple of hours, I sat on the floor by T.C. and his wife, listening to the radio. We talked about different things as we heard the unfolding, unending, shocking news. Periodically, I checked on my dad. He was either reading the three-day-old newspaper or going over by the smoking area. I was starting to notice he was smoking a little more than usual.

He didn't appear nervous, but I'm sure he was.

Chapter 12

Reality

It was approaching 2:30 p.m. on Tuesday, August 30th and I had to start getting ready for work. Word was starting to spread they were going to begin evacuating the inmates first. There was 100 percent confirmation on the levee breaks, and the 17th Street Canal levee break was on the Orleans Parish side, filling the city with floodwaters from the lake. We were only about six to seven miles from the breach, and the water outside was steadily rising. I ran over to the break room to look at our cars. The water was up to the door on my dad's car and halfway up the wheel of my car. I still had hope the waters would recede and we could get out of there, although my dad's car wasn't looking good.

Walking back to get dressed for work, I overheard a ranking official tell a deputy, "They only have enough food left to feed the inmates one meal a day for another day or two, max." I would soon find out the warehouse and the main kitchen for the entire facility were completely flooded and unusable. Making my way up the stairs, I saw a door open to what I thought was a maintenance area. This area was between the second and third floors of the building. This was the first time I'd been in that area. Voices piqued my curiosity.

One of them sounded like my supervisor's, Nurse Robert. He's the nurse supervisor for the Psychiatric Department and is a commissioned deputy for the sheriff's office.

I crept into the dark, stinky area. This building has had about 75 years of hard use, and it looked like it. At the entrance, there are some metal stairs that go down about six feet to the floor. A few huge steel tanks stand to the right with a wall directly to the left. About 20 feet past that, the area opens up slightly. To the left, ahead about 30 feet, there are double doors leading to an area I never knew existed. Robert and a couple of deputies were there.

"Hey Robert, I was on my way up to the 10th floor, and I thought I heard your voice. What is this place?"

In a matter-of-fact tone he replied, "In short, this is the main plumbing and waste management area. Pretty nasty, huh?" As soon as he said that, a little rat scurried down a ledge and into a hole in the wall.

Pointing behind him, I said, "What's behind those doors?"

"That's the outside of the building. Come check it out." We had to step up on a wooden crate and when the doors swung open, we were standing outside on top of the second floor roof of the House of Detention, directly above the cafeteria area. It took me a moment to realize we were on a flat roof area. A huge extension expanded out around the entire building in the shape of an upside down letter "T". The inmates' recreational area was to the right of the center part and barbed wire went all around the perimeter. The area was filled with three or four feet of water, making it look like a big cesspool.

We walked around the south portion and I could see the water level and my car pretty well. My dad's car definitely had water in it now, and the water level was up to the bottom of my door. It looked like it was just a matter of time now before they both were swamped.

"Son of a bitch!" I exclaimed.

Robert turned to me, "What's wrong, Gavin?"

"My dad's car is about gone and mine's next. Look, my car is the only one in the lot that doesn't have water in it yet!"

"Yeah, you might as well kiss that baby goodbye. Too bad. It looks pretty new."

"Yeah, I've only had it a little over a year ... damn!"

We examined the damage around the entire building. Hundreds of cars littered the streets. Even if my car miraculously survived, we weren't going to be able to drive out of there. It was clear things had worsened. We were in crisis mode. Wiping the sweat from my face, I took one last look at my car, then the brilliant sky and a few fires burning in the distance.

I told Nurse Robert I was going upstairs and went back through the doors. When I closed the doors it was nearly pitch black. I could see the faintest light shining around the wall by the metal stairs. I had visions of rats dropping on me and gnawing on my head or something. I quickly navigated to the metal stairs and out of the area.

The stairwell from there to the 10th floor was extremely hot. Even the walls were "sweating." The eighth and ninth floor inmates chanted and rattled the bars loudly. Those floors held disciplinary and some high-profile inmates. Those individuals tend to manipulate the system and always try to get their way. When they're caught in their little games, they are sent to the "hole" as punishment with no television or "store" [commissary] privileges. The hole is where inmates go who get out of line, fight or get caught doing something they're not supposed to. The best way to describe it would be like sending your kid to his or her room for punishment, but in this case they would be in the room the size of a closet with bars instead of a door.

The 10th floor was pretty quiet when I got there, which was quite different from the day before. Nurses Cecilia and Urban were putting medical charts in garbage bags.

"Whatcha' doin'?" I asked.

Hurried, Cecilia said, "Robert just sent word and said to get all the charts together and the medications because they will be moving the inmates soon."

I just saw Robert and he didn't say anything. "Where are they sending them?"

"Either Hunts or Angola." Angola is the Louisiana State Penitentiary — one of the roughest prisons in the country.

"When?" I asked.

"Soon. Grab a bag and give us a hand," Cecilia said.

After about 10 minutes, I remembered the inmates up there needed their medications. "What about med pass?" I asked. Both Cecilia and Urban recalled their duties.

"Damn. Gavin, why don't you start packing while Urban and I finish this?" Cecilia said.

"Did anybody count the narcotics yet?" I asked.

Urban handed me the lock box key and said, "Why don't you do it real quick, if you feel the need."

"Hey y'all, I'm gonna go find Robert and see if I can pack a few days worth of meds so we don't have to do it every shift, especially if they get moved."

Nurse Urban pointed out that a lot of the psychiatric meds couldn't be in the heat for too long. "Don't pack any Depakote (for bipolar disorder) or any gel cap pills. Can y'all think of any others?"

"I'll grab the drug book and look up as many as I can." *Great. Just when I thought I might have an easy night, I get slammed.* I ran down the stairs to try and catch Robert by the mezzanine. He wasn't there, so I went to the second floor to see if anyone had seen him. Nurse Yolanda said she thought he was in his father -inlaw's Orleans-accented voice say, "Who's that?"

After announcing myself, I was told to come in. "Yes, sir. I'm looking for Robert. Have you seen him?"

He boomed back, "Robert, come here." After about 15 seconds, Robert opened the door while wiping his face with a towel.

"Hey Gav, what's up?"

"We're up on 10 packing meds and getting the charts together. Is it all right if we get a few days' of meds just in case the inmates get moved by morning?"

Robert looked at his father-in-law and then at me and shrugged his shoulder saying, "Y'all do whatever you want — at this point I don't really care."

"All right. Will do." And with that, I hiked back up the sweltering stairwell to the 10th floor.

When I got there, I looked out over the city for a minute. We were surrounded by water for as far as I could see, but I couldn't tell where it was pouring in from. Parts of the 17th Street Canal could be seen from my building, but I couldn't see where the break in the levee was. One of the St. Bernard deputies had a radio and was sitting in the file room right across from the medical office.

"You mind turning that radio up?" someone asked.

Almost simultaneously I also heard, "Hey Gavin, what did Robert say?"

"We can do whatever we want. He doesn't care," I replied.

I found about three or four medications we use that are sensitive to heat and alerted the other two nurses. When they finished what they were doing, we packed the meds for about an hour and a half, adjusting for the heat-sensitive meds. During this time, I asked Urban about J.W.

"What's up with our little Elvis — J.W. Is he alive?"

"I think they just tried to bring him by boat, but Charity wasn't accepting anybody — they're under water as well." "What? Where is he now?" I asked.

"I think Dr. Marcus was monitoring him. I'm not sure. They think he was bottoming out (dangerously low blood pressure) from taking too much Thorazine." Thorazine is an older anti-psychotic medication that can cause dangerously low blood pressures when taken in excess.

J.W. is so disturbed he was on a pretty high dose. Coupled with the fact he fell and cut his head, he was probably going to have this problem eventually. Of course, it had to happen in the middle of this disastrous hurricane with no way to get him to the hospital.

"I hope you're right, Urban. I really don't want to deal with that situation. I have to keep an eye on my dad."

Nurse Urban asked, "Hey Gavin, how old is your dad anyways?"

"Eighty three years young; but if you ask him he will bet you that you can't guess his age."

"Why do say that?"

Laughing a little I replied, "Something to do with magic Sun-Chlorella tablets, his fountain of youth. When you see him ask him how old he is. You'll get a laugh."

We all sat around for a little while listening to the radio. The news was getting worse and worse. The gloominess in the radio announcer's voice became strangely hypnotic: "There are reports of devastation all over the city... gas lines are starting to rupture, causing numerous fires. The water is continuing to pour into the city... downtown New Orleans looks like a nuclear bomb went off... shards of glass everywhere downtown... the Central Business District is covered with glass and debris. Many of the hotel windows downtown are blown out... drapes and sheets just hanging out of the windows... and ... dead bodies floating in flood waters! We have reports of people calling 911 and our radio station for help from their attics..."

Cecilia cut in, "This is horrible! I can't imagine being stuck in an attic during the storm. And in this heat!" After a few seconds of silence, she got up. "I'm going to pass out these meds. I can't listen to this anymore."

Urban and I looked at each other, nodded our heads in unison, and got up to pass out medications.

On the med pass, some inmates asked us what was going on. A couple of them said they could hear the radio but couldn't understand what was being said. The television didn't work and you could see nervousness on their faces.

"What's going on? Why we only got one sandwich today? We need water too. We haven't gotten any water today. Water, please! What's going to happen to us?"

I decided to get everyone's attention. "Listen up guys! We're surrounded by water. Some of the levees have collapsed and water is pouring into the city."

Interrupting me at times, inmates yelled out things like, "I'm supposed to roll-out tomorrow (roll-out means get released)," or "I need to call my people."

"Hold up guys, hear me out. The phones don't work, and there is nowhere to roll out to. You'll be evacuated soon. I don't know when. We're low on food and water..."

They all started yelling and chattering and asking all kinds of questions I couldn't answer. I finished passing meds on the tier, and then I had to go down to the seventh floor, since that's where we keep some of the chronic psychiatric inmates. Those people are schizophrenics, bi-polars, psychotics, or otherwise seriously mentally ill. Some are homeless and others have families but have been disowned. It's pretty sad to see, and I try to do what I can for them. Most of them are arrested for penny-ante stuff like obstruction of a public sidewalk, trespassing, sleeping in a public park, public drunkenness, and things of that nature. The laws in New Orleans are capriciously enforced, and those people are easy targets. At least 90 percent of them are African-American and many have a history of alcohol or drug abuse. It is a common occurrence that in the city – if you're a black male and look a certain way, you have a good chance of getting arrested numerous times. It's sad.

I went down to the seventh floor, and it was hot as Hell there. Many of those guys were lying in all kinds of positions on their mattresses on the floor. Family members, staff, and friends. Since we were running on generators, the fans weren't operating. The heat was stifling, and I could see the exhaustion on their faces. There were only two toilets everyone had to share, and there was one grimy, antiquated shower at the beginning of the tier for everyone to use.

The newer part of the facility across the street had air conditioning and a modernized set-up. The main administrative building also housed federal and illegal alien inmates. The building has many floors and is as tall as the HOD building I was in.

One of the regular inmates on the seventh floor, K.R., saw me coming down the tier. "Hey nurse, hey nurse... you got my meds?"

"Hang on K, I'll get them to you in a minute." After walking the length of the tier and getting everyone's attention, I told them the same thing I told the inmates on the 10th floor. The reaction was similar and so were the questions. Ignoring most, I passed the medications out, explaining to them why certain meds were not given. I'm not really sure if they understood or not, but I tried to give them the courtesy of telling them why I was doing what I was doing.

After finishing the medication pass, I went back to the 10th floor. Cecelia was gone, and Urban and I each grabbed a mop and mopped the medical office and the surrounding walkways, in case we had any emergencies.

Normally, Urban works the "graveyard" shift from 11 p.m. to 7:30 a.m. He is a very interesting character. I don't think I can describe him very well, but he's a very knowledgeable person and an outstanding nurse. He was helping us out on this shift, which I greatly appreciated. Once we finished cleaning up (we never really finished — too much water) we started talking about his family and mine. He wasn't sure if his father evacuated or not. He brought his mother to the facility with him and she was a godsend. She is a diminutive Latino lady who appears to have Bell's palsy or something, since the left side of her face droops. She's extremely feisty and has a very strong Central American accent which is at times difficult to understand.

After we talked for an hour or so, Urban went back downstairs, and I asked him to keep an eye on my dad. I don't know why I was extra worried about my father, but I was.

Around that time, Nurse Favis came to the 10th floor. We usually work together on the evening shift. She apologized for coming up late, saying she had lost track of time. She had her daughter with her, and she was trying to entertain her and keep an eye on her. I told her not too worry about her tardiness, and for the next couple hours it was relatively quiet. We had only one fistfight and no one was hurt badly. I gave her an update of what we did with the medical charts and the medication pass.

The highlight of being on the 10th floor was J.W.'s return. I don't really know what happened, but the doctors sent him back, and we were to check his vital signs every hour for the next 48 hours or as long as he was here. They must have stabilized him long enough to feel he was all right. When he saw me, he greeted me with his usual, "Hey, Dad!" It never gets old to me. I always laugh a little on the inside. We're basically the same age and it's funny he keeps calling me "Dad." Sometimes I try to imagine how it must be to be out of touch with reality. With the situation at hand, ignorance may truly have been bliss.

We decided to shuffle some of the inmates around and keep J.W. in a cell by the front of the north tier by himself. I wasn't completely comfortable he was out of the woods, health-wise.

We thought if we kept him by himself, maybe he would stay calm. We told him not to play in the dirty water on the floor, and if he did, we would place him in five-point restraints, which are used for inmates who are acting bizarre, hostile, or suicidal. This is the best method I have seen to control an inmate. It is amazing how fast they change their minds about being suicidal or violent. It doesn't always work, but usually it does. Restraints are used because every inmate cannot be watched at all times. If something happens to that inmate or another inmate, the sheriff's office is ultimately responsible.

We got J.W. settled in, and I notified the deputy that a couple of the tiers were low on drinking water. The deputy said he knew and had notified the Watch Office. "They're just gonna have to wait. Nothing I can do about it right now." When the inmates were told this, they complained loudly.

It was just about dark outside as the sun slipped under the orange-blue skyline. Plumes of smoke blended with the darkening horizon. Not a single streetlight could be seen in the distance.

Taking one last look at our cars, I could see the roof of my dad's car and I couldn't really tell, but it looked like the water was about midway up my door. Every car in the lot was flooded. They looked like matchbox cars in a large muddy puddle. Favis came over and pointed out her car. All I could see was the back section of the roof.

"I'm so glad that piece of junk got flooded. Now I can get somethin' else. Always givin' me trouble."

I interjected, "Not me — my car is only a year old. I'm sure I'm gonna get screwed on my insurance."

It was strangely calm and quiet. We only had light down the hallways of the 10th floor and the tiers. The two bathrooms on the 10th floor for the medical staff and security to use weren't working.

As you might imagine, the toilet was not pleasant, and that's putting it mildly. I hate to say it, but I urinated in the sink. The circumstances made us all do things we wouldn't have normally done.

It seemed like every time I sat down to listen to the radio, the announcers sounded just flat-out deflated. After 20 or so minutes of listening to it, I asked Favis if I could go down a little early and check on my dad. She pleasantly replied, "Sure, I've got it up here." It was amazing to see how my coworkers kept their calm and pulled together as the situation worsened.

"Come get me if you need something; and don't forget to check on J.W. See ya later," I said.

I felt a lot better physically that day than the day before. I only had to go up and down the stairs a few times. It was still inferno-hot and completely dark in the stairwell. Passing up the mezzanine, I heard some voices but decided to keep on moving.

I made my way through the doorway and onto the second floor. A few stragglers walked around, but most people were sleeping or listening to the radio. Some talked about the other buildings in the facility that had lost power completely and were under four to eight feet of water. Some inmates were trying to escape, but none were successful, as far as we knew.

I saw Dr. Marcus; he told me that IPC and Templeman buildings I, II, III, and IV were completely swamped with water. "I was sleeping on a couch in TP I and II last night and when I woke up and sat up my legs were in water. We had to move to the third floor and then all you could hear was the rattle of bars and hateful chorus of the inmates, 'Kill the white mother fuckers! Kill the white mother fuckers! Kill the …'"

Dr. Marcus had valiantly moved from building-to-building in the water by swimming or floating on something. By Tuesday afternoon, he had pretty much settled at our building, the House of Detention.

I overheard all kinds of stuff while I was changing my shirt over by my mattress. My dad was sleeping, and I didn't disturb him. It was around 10 p.m., and I decided to clean up a little. I had a couple gallons of Kentwood Spring Water so I took my towel, poured some water on it and wiped my face, neck, arms, and armpits.

After putting some deodorant on, I grabbed my toothbrush and toothpaste and went to the bathroom sink near us. I tried to turn on one of the faucets, figuring that it wouldn't work, and it didn't. I poured some bottled water into a cup, put some toothpaste on my toothbrush, and brushed away. It was about this time that I noticed the bathroom stunk really, really badly. The overuse was starting to show. There was a trash all over the floor, and I could tell there wasn't any concern to keep the bathroom somewhat clean.

I made the decision at that point that I wasn't going to eat until I was absolutely starving so I could avoid going to the bathroom as much as possible. It dawned on me trying to convince my dad to do the same would be a difficult task.

I settled in to my mattress and put on my portable DVD player and started to watch the movie, "Left Behind," a movie about the End Times with references to the Bible's Book of Revelations. How appropriate. I had been watching the movie for only a little while when the whole building went completely dark. A few kids and others screamed, some laughed, and gradually a few flashlights flickered on. About five minutes later, the ranking official in charge of the building walked in and with his booming voice announced, "Everybody listen up! The generator is flooded, and we are out of power!"

As he talked, two deputies walked in with crowbars and shotguns. They ordered everyone who was near a window (that was us) to move their things so they could break the windows to try and get some air to circulate. I woke my dad and helped him sit up.

Sounding completely confused and startled he asked, "What the hell is going on? Why is it so dark in here?"

"The power is out, Dad. The generator is flooded," I explained. "Get up. Hurry up! We've got to move our stuff away from the window so they can bust them out." "Do what?" He was confused.

"Just get up and stand over there."

While we moved our things, I could hear the boss saying, "Everybody stay calm. We're making arrangements to evacuate everyone. For safety reasons, we'll be moving the inmates first."

I could hear people starting to complain, but it made sense to me to move the inmates first. "Everyone will be evacuated! Please be patient! That's it!"

The deputies started to smash the thick windows with the crowbars as the boss walked away, the shattered glass falling in small pieces to the floor. The window to my left started to crack open, and the other deputy struck another window. Further away, Corporal Mitchell came up and stood next to me, but I didn't really pay much attention to him.

Then, BANG! I heard a gun go off and a sharp pain hit my right leg. My heart felt like it was in my stomach. The deputy jumped and almost dropped the crowbar on his head. It was so dark in there that no one but the deputy, Corporal Mitchell, and I knew that the gun wasn't aimed at the window.

After looking at the deputy, I grabbed the candle off of the nearby table and shined it in the direction of my leg and saw that it was bleeding. I looked over to my right and could see a horrified look on Corporal Mitchell's face.

I cried out, "What the fuck happened?!"

"The gun accidentally went off in my hand. Holy Shit! I almost shot my foot off, man."

"You almost shot your foot? You almost shot my fucking leg off man! You trying to kill me or what?"

Half whispering he said, "Shhhhhh! Man ... it was an accident. I thought the safety was on. This mutha' fucker has a hair trigger on it!" Simultaneously, we both looked at the floor with his flashlight and we could see where the shot put a black mark a couple of inches wide. The piece of the floor must have hit my leg.

"You got my heart racing!"

"Mine too. Damn! That was close." I grabbed a towel from out of my bag and wiped my leg while Corporal Mitchell explained to me this shotgun was actually an air gun used for impact and did not use bullets or shells.

Thank God for that or I might be a one-legged nurse! It took about five minutes of whacking the window to get most of the glass out. It was after 11 p.m., and the second floor was alive and kicking.

You could hear frantic conversations and tension in people's voices. We got some brooms and dustpans so we could clean up the glass on the floor. Using a couple of flashlights and a candle, we picked up the bigger chunks by hand, trying not to cut ourselves in the process. Once the area was swept up, we started to put our stuff back in its spot. Deputy Jeanne and her boyfriend had a couple candles lit on the table we had moved back by the wall. One had an image of what appeared to be a Spanish-looking Jesus Christ on it. It was made of glass and about a foot tall. It lit up the area quite well, considering how dark it was.

I got my dad's mattress situated against the wall again and put the sheet back on it for him. I turned to tell him to lie back down but he wasn't there. T.C. was over by his spot. I asked him where my dad was, and he said he saw him walking towards the visitors' area. I went over there to find him sitting at the end of the walkway smoking a cigarette. "Hey, your bed is made and your stuff is back where it was, okay? You all right?"

Shining the flashlight in his direction, I could see he was a little concerned, but he would never admit it to me. "Oh, yeah, Son. I'll be over there in a minute."

It was also apparent he wanted to be alone so I said, "I'm gong back over to fix my bed. See you in a minute." Walking away, I looked back and noticed he was lighting up another cigarette, confirming that he was becoming increasingly uneasy with the situation — just like the rest of us.

Back by our spot, I put a sheet on my mattress and Deputy Kite asked, "Is your daddy all right?"

"I guess so. I just think he's out of his element, and he doesn't quite know what to think of all this. I'm a little worried about him."

"If there is anything I can do just let me know."

"I appreciate that. Thanks."

For the next few minutes, I sat quietly and listened to everything going on around me. My mind was starting to race. My dad came back and gingerly laid down next to me on his mattress.

"Everything all right, Pops?"

"Think we'll be going home soon?"

"I'm not sure, but I hope so."

"I do too because I need my medicine soon. I'm gonna try and get some sleep."

Damn. I had forgotten he was running low on his medication. Coupled with his increased smoking, I worried about his health. I didn't want anything to happen to him. He deserved better; we all did. With all the horrible things I was hearing on the radio, I was glad he was with me, but not in the jail with me.

"Good night, Dad."

"Good night, Son."

I fixed a stare at the candle on the table. The Jesus image on the candle looked right at me. I have never been ultrareligious or anything, but just looking at that lit image had a calming effect.

Everyone around us started to settle down a little bit. The bathroom was only about 30 feet from our mattresses, and people were going in and out at a steady pace. In the night, there was one problem: the bathroom had only a sliding latch on it and no doorstopper. When someone would go in, they would close the door, slamming it loudly.

It was annoying at night to be asleep and then abruptly awakened with the slamming door. Some people were considerate and closed the door slowly, except the younger teenagers. It was like they were trying to make the loudest noise by having the door slam behind them.

Chapter 13

Frustration

We'd been trapped for almost four days. It was after midnight, and my dad had fallen asleep, which made me feel a little better. For as late as it was, it was extremely hot and muggy, like sauna hot. A hint of a warm breeze would come through the jagged window from time to time, but it didn't do much good.

When I laid my head down on the pillow, I could see outside to the sky through a small part of the window. Words can't describe how I felt. The stars in the sky were truly amazing — billions and billions of bright stars. With all the lights out, you could see the night sky in unbelievable detail. Chills went down my entire body. I have been out in the countryside before and have never seen that many stars at night.

I was drawn to it. I got up off my mattress and carefully stuck my head out of the narrow, glass-splintered window. There were still some glass pieces sticking out of the window and I really didn't feel like getting one of my ears cut off. It was phenomenal though, like the Milky Way was blanketing New Orleans: clear, crisp and sparkling. I felt the power of the universe upon us. For what we were going through, all those stars shining made me believe there was a higher power looking over us.

With the devastation surrounding us, the beautiful midnight sky was truly something to behold.

I will never forget the feeling of peace and awe and wonder I had at that moment.

Then suddenly, pop, pop, POW... Pop, POW POW! Gunshots pierced the serene silence.

Stunned, I quickly but carefully pulled my head back in through the jagged window. That was the first time in my life I had ever heard live gunfire close by like that. And it didn't stop there. It seemed like every 15 minutes or so, for the next couple of hours, I heard a gunshot here, two or three there.

Bang, bang POW POW! Pop POW POW POW!

I didn't know if they were coming from the police, deputies, civilians, or what. This was all starting to feel like a bad movie. I was afraid for my dad and myself.

We obviously were in survival mode. Lying there, I looked out the shattered window, my mind racing. I couldn't fall asleep. I wasn't sure, but it felt like my air mattress was starting to sink just as our hopes were. I grabbed the flashlight and looked under and around the mattress and checked the air hole, but didn't see anything wrong.

If I had to guess, it was after two o'clock in the morning by then, and I hadn't gotten any sleep. Lying back down, I took a few deep breaths to try to help me go to sleep. It must have worked but before I knew it, "KABOOM!" A huge explosion went off that scared me right off my half-deflated mattress.

What the hell was that?

It was still dark so I reached for my cell phone and turned it on to see what the time was. For as loud as that was, I was grateful my dad stayed asleep. It was 5:12 a.m., and my phone still had no signal. It was still dark and the stars were still brilliantly twinkling through the broken window.

It was Heaven and Hell all at once.

I had to go to the bathroom, so I turned my flashlight on and navigated my way there. After carefully closing the door, an eyepopping stench smacked me in the face. Now the plumbing didn't work. I put the flashlight under my left armpit and pulled my shirt up over my nose and took a pee. Then I went back to my bed and attempted to get some sleep. As soon as I lay down, my dad woke up and told me he had to go to the bathroom, so I told him I would go with him. I planned to show him how bad it was and maybe he could wait.

"I got it, Son."

Whispering, I asked him, "Number one or number two?"

"What?"

"Come on, it's dark and I'll help you with the flashlight." Looking around real quick, I grabbed the sheet off of my bed and brought it with us.

"What's that for?" he asked.

"I'll let you know in a minute."

After almost tripping over a couple of people we made it to the bathroom. Once inside I shined the flashlight on the toilets so he could see the piles of human waste.

"Goddamn. I'm not going in there!"

"Look, Dad, I'm gonna tear this sheet and cover the sink. You can sit on top and go in there. It's better than the alternative."

"I guess so, Son." The sheet was worn anyway, and I didn't want to risk either one of us getting sick from the heaps of urine-soaked feces in the bathroom. I tore a piece just big enough to cover the sink. After helping him up on the sink, I walked to the back on the side of the bathroom and grabbed a roll of toilet paper for him. I walked over by the door so he could do his business.

There was a shattered window in the bathroom, and after he was done I took the sheet, tied it up and threw it out the window into the water, which was at least ten feet high. We both looked at each other and broke out into laughter.

What else could we do?

I told him to wait a second and I would be right back. I went back to our spot, grabbed my towel and a bottle of water, and brought it back to the bathroom. I told him to hold his hands out and cup them and I poured the water in his hands, and then used the towel to dry his hands. Once we were done, we walked back, by flash-light, to our area.

It was after 6 a.m. by now and some sunlight was just beginning to creep through the broken window by our spot. It was extremely hot for that time of the day, and I knew it was going to be a very long, hot, humid one. I told my dad I was not going to eat much so I could avoid the bathroom as much as I possible, hoping he'd take the hint. I took a couple sips of water and encouraged him to do the same. He did and laid back down. I told him I had a few pairs of shorts with me if he wanted a pair to wear.

"You got something to fit me?"

"Not really, but you can leave the top button open and I think that might work." I had a baggy pair with a drawstring at the top that he could probably fit into.

"Here you go, Pops." He sat back and took his pants off. Thank God he had boxer briefs on, and it was still early in the morning. He put the shorts on saying, "Ah ... that's better. You wear these, Son?" They were plaid shorts that could be used for swimming.

Jokingly, I replied, "You never know, we might have to swim out of here."

He turned to me real quick and said, "What?"

"I'm kidding, Dad. I'll be right back. I'm going to look out the window to see how our cars are doing."

While I was on the way to the break room, I noticed there were a lot more people sleeping in the big hallway than the night before. It was dark and I needed my flashlight to maneuver through it. I wondered about the batteries. As you might expect, our cars were surrounded by a watery grave. What little hope I had held out was crushed in the bright morning sun. The water was now three-quarters of the way up my window and obviously over the hood of the car. Cars that I could see the day before were no longer visible. The water was a dark brownish color and had what looked like oil slicks covering most of it.

I was really numb at this point, wondering how Lora was doing and realizing now I didn't have a car and neither did my dad. We're both very independent people, but it was clear we would be joined at the hip for a while. A minute or two later, I heard what sounded like the engine of a flat boat. After watching the boat go around the building, I went back by my dad and told him the bad news. "Well, Dad, you want the bad news or the bad news?"

"What?"

"You can barely see the roof of your car and the water is three-quarters of the way up the window of my car."

"Well, when the water goes down, maybe she'll start up!"

"Your car is completely submerged in the water. She ain'tstartin'." I could see he didn't want to accept this and sat there absorbing it in silence.

"When are we going home?"

I paused before answering because I could feel myself starting to get frustrated and angry. I could see he didn't really comprehend the severity of the situation. I had to give it to him straight. "Dad, listen, we don't know how your place is. I don't know how my place is. We need to get the hell out of here first and foremost. Forget about going home any time soon. Let's try and get out of here first."

"But the storm is over. When the water goes down we'll just catch a ride."

At this point, I could see he really believed this would be over soon. I tried to explain, "The levees have collapsed, Dad. There's water pouring into the city from the lake, maybe the river... I don't know. The water isn't going down any time soon. I'll try to find what's going on in the next couple of hours. I'll let you know when I find something out."

The smell of diesel gas had filled the room. I decided to go investigate. It was after 7 a.m., and no one was in the Watch Office. I heard someone say all the deputies and ranking officials were having a meeting. I ran up to the 10th floor to take a look at the city.

There were only a few people up there. Nurse Donna was just finishing up her shift. "What's up Gavin? Why are you up here so early?"

"I came up to take a look at the city. How was last night?" "Not too bad. Typical stuff."

I went over to the south side to look out the window. The sky was cloudless: beautiful, clear, and hopeful. It was strange that since the hurricane passed through we hadn't had a cloud in the sky.

It was as if we were starting over. But there wasn't any breeze at all, either. I saw a couple military helicopters in the distance. When I went to the north side, I saw a massive plume of black smoke flowing from the east, like ink flowing up into the placid heavens.

"Jesus! Did y'all see that smoke over there?" Before they could answer, I said, "I heard a huge explosion this morning around five o'clock. That must be where the smoke is coming from."

Nobody really acknowledged me. It was as if we were helplessly watching Rome burn. "Hey Donna, did you see that smoke out there?"

"What smoke? Where?"

"Come see. Over there."

"Damn! Where the hell is that coming from?"

"I have no idea, but I heard an explosion a couple of hours ago so I guess that's where it's coming from. This is turning into Baghdad West."

After about 10 minutes of looking at the worsening situation, I went back downstairs to see if I could find out where that diesel smell was coming from. When I got to the second floor, there were more people walking around. I saw Nurse Favis. "You smell that?" I asked.

"Yeah, smells like diesel gas or something," she said, with a funny look on her face.

In unison, we asked, "Where's that coming from?"

Laughing as I walked away, I said, "When I find out I'll let you know."

"All right, G."

I finally found Nurse Robert and asked him about the smell. He said, "I was told that the flood water overflowed the generator and went down the exhaust pipes, and that's where it's coming from."

"Sounds right to me. Thanks. Hey, are you going up to the 10th floor today?"

"Nope. I'm pretty much a deputy from here on out."

"By the way, when are we getting out of here?" I asked. "Hopefully soon."

Unfortunately, that would be a recurring theme. I went back over to see my dad. "Hey, Dad. That smell is coming ..." It didn't look like he understood me too well so I didn't want to confuse him anymore. "Don't worry about it, Dad. Just hang in there. They're working on getting us out of here."

"Okay, Son. I'm a little hungry."

Grabbing my bag, I took some granola bars out to show him. "I have peanut butter, oatmeal raisin, chocolate chip ..."

"Chocolate chip!"

"Here you go. Do you want some water or lemonade?" I asked.

"A cup of coffee would be great."

"We don't have any power to make any coffee, Pops. Here — drink a few sips of water."

It was approaching 8 a.m., and the heat was already starting to be a factor. The bathroom odor had made its way around the second floor. We were only 10 yards or so from the bathroom, and it seemed like every other person was letting the door slam. My dad said, "I'll be right back," and started to walk toward the visitors' area, I assumed to catch a smoke. A few kids ran around making noise as other people sat around listening to the radio or talking among themselves. I saw T.C. and his wife adjusting the antenna on their radio, so I made my way over to them. "What's up T.C.?"

"Hey G, whatcha' say?"

About that time the radio announcer was saying something about looters. "We have people running around looting downtown New Orleans. We have reports of an NOPD officer being shot in the back of the head by a looter. He's in critical condition at West Jefferson Medical Center ... the suspect is also there with injuries as well."

T.C. and I exchanged wide-eyed looks and just shook our heads. "Man, this is crazy, Gavin."

Two days after the storm and cops were being shot!

"Pretty unbelievable. I wonder what the hell is next?"

We turned our attention back to the radio as the announcer continued, "There are areas of the city where the water looks like it's boiling. The gas lines are rupturing and igniting numerous fires around the metro area ... the fire department is stretched so thin they're letting some of the fires just burn. The water pressure is almost non-existent ... no part of the city is exempt from the fires. We have families just standing on corners looking dazed ... thousands upon thousands of people with no food or water ... BODIES floating in the water near the Superdome ... chaos at the New Orleans Convention Center with reports of gun battles, fighting, rapes ..." and so on. A horrid picture.

Where was our mayor? Our governor? Our president? Was help coming?

I sat there wondering what was going to happen to us. The inmates were riotously loud and it was getting hotter by the minute.

I got up and told T.C., "I'll be back in a little while." Walking back over to my spot, I felt tears welling up in my eyes. I couldn't help it. I don't know why, I just had this sudden feeling of complete helplessness. My emotions were childlike. Images flashed through my mind like a high-speed movie. I remembered, as a kid, my dad being so much older, and I would worry he would die or not be there for some reason or the other.

After my parents divorced when I was eight, it took me a long time to get past this fear. My mother eventually remarried, and I have to say my dad was there for me every step of the way. Now here we were in this nightmare.

So this is what it's come to?

What did we do to deserve this?

Would he die here?

Was this it?

Here's a man who was born in the 1920s, grew up in the Great Depression, made it through World War II, and was a fairly well-known jazz musician in the city. He'd played with greats like Louie Prima and Al Hirt. He had started a long career at the world-famous Roosevelt Hotel in New Orleans and then the Blue Room in the Fairmont Hotel for over 35 years, and had even been on the Tonight Show with Harry Connick Jr.

After 83 years of a pretty good life, he was in one of the worst situations ever. It's hard for me to convey exactly what was going on in my head. The bottom line was my dad is a good man and had been very good to me, and I just didn't want anything to happen to him. Those feelings poured out like a volcano erupting. It was then I steeled my resolve to do whatever it took to keep him safe and his mind right. I knew this would be one of the greatest challenges of my life. I had to figure out a way to get him to understand what we were facing without upsetting or scaring him.

As all this was going through my mind, I saw my dad drop a cigarette butt on the floor and step on it. Luckily, I don't think anyone saw him. I quickly got up and met him as he walked toward me. "Dad, you can't do that."

"Look, Son, stop telling me what to do. I'm still your father!" Same old Dad, thank goodness.

"Don't give me a damn reason to say anything. Stay over in the designated spot until you're done smoking, please," I replied.

He mumbled "all right" as he walked away from me and sat down on his mattress.

I looked at him for a minute or so and then walked over. "Hey look, Dad. I'm sorry if you think I keep telling you what to do; it's just that in here we've gotta follow the rules with no exceptions. We're in here with a bunch of other folks, and they're on edge."

"All right. I didn't realize what I was doing until you said something. Sorry, I'm just ready to go."

"Me too, Buddy. As soon as I find anything out, I'll let you know."

As he turned his head to look out the window, the bathroom door slammed again. My dad yelled, "Why the hell does everyone keep slamming the door?"

"I haven't got a clue, Dad. I'm gonna go get some paper and put a sign on the door."

I went over to the second floor clinic. It was still dark as a coalmine. I asked if anyone was in there and got no response. I went back to get a flashlight so I could find some paper, tape, and a pen, then I went back to my half-inflated mattress and made two signs – one for the front of the door and one for the back of the door.

They both read, "PLEASE DON'T SLA.M THE DOOR!" Simple and to the point.

After taping the signs to each side of the door, a little old black lady came up and thanked me. "Thank you Son ... I hope this works. That damn banging is really getting on my nerves. Really unnecessary — all that bangin', you know?"

"You're welcome, ma'am. Spread the word. Maybe people will be more considerate."

I went over to the doorway by the recreational area. Before I got there, I saw Nurse/Deputy Robert and a few other people going through the stairwell that leads to the 10th floor. Curious, I followed after them, lagging behind. To my surprise, they went through the door at the mezzanine level. I followed and when I got in there they were on the roof area again. I went out and saw there were a few people walking around surveying the area.

I asked Robert what was going on and he said, "They're startin' to evacuate the inmates to the Broad Street Bridge, and then upstate."

Even more curious, I asked, "Where? To Angola or something?"

"Angola, Hunts, all over the South, probably."

"What building are they starting with?"

"TP I, II, III, and IV first, then probably OPP (Orleans Parish Prison). I'm not really sure."

"When will they move our building?"

Robert turned to me with a blank, uncertain look on his face. "Probably last, because we're on the second floor and the water hasn't gotten up to our floor yet, unlike some of the other buildings."

I looked down at the water surrounding our building. I wondered how high it had to get before they moved us. It was getting close to 11 a.m., and the day was becoming a real scorcher. With the oppressively humid August weather and no sign of a cloud in the sky to protect us, we were getting the full brunt of the sun beating down.

I stared at the thick smoke coming right over our building. It appeared to be coming from the Mississippi River area. When I walked back downstairs, I asked a couple people if they knew where the smoke was coming from, but no one did. There was an older African-American gentleman sitting by the break room, listening to the radio.

"Excuse me, sir. Have you heard anything about a huge fire or explosion?"

"Can't say that I have, Son."

"Thanks anyway."

I went back over by my dad to see how he was doing. He was lying down, drenched in sweat and looking overheated.

"You feelin' all right, Dad?"

"I don't know. I feel a little dizzy. I don't know if it's from the heat or what."

"Do you want me to check your blood pressure?" He started to sit up, then immediately laid back down.

"Don't move. I can check it while you're lying down. I'll be right back."

I hustled over to the second floor clinic, grabbed a blood pressure cuff and stethoscope and took his blood pressure. It was a little elevated and his pulse was too. I helped him to his feet and took his blood pressure again. It was still mildly elevated, but his pulse was bounding at 104 beats a minute. This was possibly a sign of mild dehydration, so I explained this to him and got him to drink a bottle of water.

Helping him lay back down, I told him to relax and grabbed my pillow and fanned him with it. "That's not necessary, Son. You don't have to."

Not thinking twice, I said, "I don't mind. Hey, how many blood pressure pills do you have left?"

"Five or so."

I told him I went upstairs earlier to the clinic to see if we had his type of blood pressure medicine, but we didn't. "Don't worry," I told him. "I'll talk to one of the doctors to see if there is something comparable that we can substitute."

After a couple minutes of fanning my dad, I told him to drink more water at the first sign of dizziness and to slack off on the smoking.

"I haven't been smoking that much," he said.

I knew he had, but I wasn't going to argue with him.

Nurse Cecelia walked by while I fanned my dad. "Is he all right?" she asked.

"Yeah, just a little hot and dizzy," I replied.

"If you need anything, let me know."

"Thanks." I fanned him for about a half-hour more until he fell asleep. I went to stand by the bathroom door to make sure no one would slam it and wake him. The smell was damn awful, but I felt I had to keep the noise down as much as I could so my dad could rest. Standing there, I tried to point out the signs to people as they came and went. especially the younger ones.

People around the room fanned themselves with whatever they could. I know I keep harping on the heat, but it was brutal. No breeze or circulation of air to speak of. I knew elderly people and infants around the city were surely dying from it. After an hour or so, I decided I needed some fresh air. On my way to the recreational area, I saw Dr. Marcus and two nurses running to the stairwell that leads to the 10th floor. There must have been some sort of emergency, but I didn't have the energy to ask.

The doorway was crowded and a sickly man sat in a wheelchair with a nasal cannula running to his nose. His oxygen tank was attached to the side of his wheelchair. I couldn't believe my eyes when he took the nasal cannula off his head and lit up a cigarette. He probably had chronic obstruction pulmonary disease or some other respiratory problem, and it was maybe 120 degrees in there, and he lit up a cigarette! We were basically stranded, and our supplies were running short. What was he thinking?

After a few seconds of watching this guy, I left to see what was going on out on the roof. Once I got up there, I noticed the number of people had swelled quite a bit. When I walked out the door, I heard a loud swooshing sound so I walked around to investigate the noise. I saw a military helicopter with a Red Cross symbol hovering right above the roof. The wind generated from the helicopter was ferocious and it felt like an oven-hot tornado. Even so, any wind felt pretty good.

After about two or three minutes of the helicopter looking like it was going to land, it dropped some water and supplies and eased straight up in the air and took off. Deputies moved the supplies back toward to the main part of the roof by the entrance door.

Whoever was on the roof was able to take some water if they needed it, so I grabbed a couple of bottles and went back down by my dad.

Some areas of the second floor were active with people and others did not have as much movement. The heat seemed to affect everyone differently. My dad was lying down looking up at the ceiling with his hands behind his head.

"Hey, Buddy, you awake?" I asked.

"Yeah. Damn door keeps slamming. Can't people see the sign?"

"You would think; it's right by the door knob. I stood over there for an hour earlier while you were sleeping so I could stop it from slamming."

He acknowledged my efforts with a smile then asked me to look at his back. "It's itching like crazy!"

When I removed his shirt I saw that he had a bad heat rash or something. "Let me go get some hydrocortisone cream to help with the itching." The second floor clinic didn't have any, so I took the stairs to the 10th floor. Winded, I stopped on the eighth floor to catch my breath. When I got to the 10th floor, I looked out the window and saw what looked like at least a dozen military helicopters in the air in a square formation. It looked like they were hovering, doing some sort of surveillance. It was strange to see the military presence, but I was glad to see them. After watching this for a few minutes, I searched the supply room and found a couple of tubes of hydrocortisone cream.

Exhausted and running on adrenaline, I eventually got back to our area just in time to see my dad trying to scratch his back with his shoe.

Moving behind him I said, "Pull your shirt up or off and I'll rub this cream on your back." I know it must have looked pretty funny, rubbing this cream on his back while his old man boobs jiggled around. I hate to knock the old man, but his man-boobs are droopy. I was snickering to myself a little bit and he heard me, "What's so funny? What's so funny?"

"This is. Rubbing cream on your back, in a jail, in sweltering heat when you could have been sitting on a couch at your sister's house in the air conditioning!"

With a half-hearted smile he said, "I guess you're right. Don't rub it in!" We both laughed as a young teenage girl walked by crinkling her nose while giving us a peculiar look. After covering his back, I told Dad to lie on his side and I would fan his back with the pillow. I fanned him for quite a while and eventually I was covered with sweat. I grabbed a chair nearby and sat down and took my shirt off, continuing to fan him until he was sound asleep. I don't really remember how long I fanned him, but the next thing I knew, I fell out the chair, landing on my right knee and elbow on my now deflated mattress.

"Ouch! Damn!" My dad didn't hear me since he was sound asleep. I got up, grabbed my towel, and wiped the sweat from my arms, chest, and face.

It looked like my dad wasn't breathing. His mouth was slightly open and he was lying on his side. I watched for about 10 more seconds and still no breath. I didn't want to wake him up if he was sleeping, but for a moment I wasn't sure. I got a sinking feeling and then a panicking feeling. Just as I was about to shake him, he took a big, deep breath through his nose and mouth, making a loud snoring noise.

I jumped back a little and breathed a sigh of relief. I don't know why I thought the worst at this moment, but I did. I took a bottle of water and my towel and try to clean myself up a little bit. Turning toward the stench factory bathroom, I saw Dr. Marcus walking toward me, holding his right hand around his wrist with his left hand. It looked as if it was totally limp or broken. I could see he was in pain, but it looked more like he was in shock.

"What happened to your hand, Doc?"

"An Epi-Pen went through my hand and it's totally numb!" An Api-Pen is an injection used when someone is having a severe asthma attack and can't breathe. It is a measured dose of epinephrine that helps open the airways so the person having the attack can breathe normally.

"How the hell did that happen?"

"We went up to the fourth or fifth floor, I really don't know, because someone was having an asthma attack from the heat. We couldn't get his condition under control. It was dark as hell on the tier. There were inmates standing all around, and when I grabbed the Epi-Pen and took the top off I almost dropped it. Luckily, or I guess in this case unluckily for me, I had the wrong end in my hand. When I went to jam the needle in his thigh, it went right through my hand."

At this point, he showed me how far the needle had gone through the other side of his hand. "It felt like a gunshot going right through my hand."

With a grimace on my face, I said, "Damn, Doc; did it hit any bones?"

"I don't believe so, but I really couldn't tell you right now because my whole hand is numb." He grabbed his wrist and started to shake his right hand. "It feels like the numbness is going up my arm."

An Epi-Pen is flush on both sides, and the needle doesn't extend out until pressure is applied to the injection. So if he couldn't see the pen, it's not surprising he accidentally injected himself.

"Is there anything I can do?"

He smiled and said, "You could help me take a leak."

I did a double take look at him, "Do what?"

He started to laugh and said, "Just kidding, Gavin!"

"Good! Because you would've been on your own there."

"No, seriously, I just need to take a nap. I haven't really slept since Monday night, and that wasn't enough sleep."

"Where's your stuff?" I asked.

"I only have a couple of things. When I left Templeman I and II, I left some stuff over there. The water was rising so fast we had to get out of there!"

"Do you have anything to sleep on?"

"Nope."

"Let me go see if I can find you a mattress."

"Oh, that's all right. I'll just sleep by you all on the floor."

"Doc, please let me try to find you something, a mattress or something. In the meantime, use my half-ass air mattress." By this point, my mattress was fairly flat, but at least I wasn't sleeping directly on the floor.

I went to the Watch Office to see if there were any mattresses left. Ms. Sandra, a control deputy, said to check with one of the ranking officials. I looked for 20 minutes or so and couldn't find a soul. I went up to the roof again and there were plenty of people up there. I saw Robert, and he said he didn't know where I could get a mattress for the doctor. As he was walking away I asked, "Any word on leaving yet?"

"I heard maybe tomorrow morning if not sooner."

"Oh, that's great! I'll see you later."

I decided to go try and clean up a little now that I had a chance. My dad was still sleeping and but only taking a breath every 10 seconds or so. Maybe he had sleep apnea. I still felt the need to watch him for a minute or so to make sure he was breathing okay. I couldn't escape the steady paranoia that I was feeling. I didn't want my dad to die in there.

I took my bottle of water and poured some of it over my head and onto my towel. I scrubbed my head and wiped off my arms and neck. I looked up into the mirror and saw that my hair looked like I stuck my finger in a light socket. I took my hand and ran it through my hair and to my dismay, I had quite a few hairs in my hand. *Great! I'm gonna start losing my hair on top of everything else.* I did it again with the same result. I remembered my longtime friend, Ron, telling me, "Don't worry big boy, when you turn 33, it'll start coming out!" Well, I turned 33 the month before the hurricane.

Dammit! Standing there with no shirt on, hair in my hand, no real shower in five days, and a sewer for a bathroom, I walked out not feeling so good. This was getting to me.

After a few minutes of self-pity, I changed my shirt and put some shorts on. It was past my time to go up to work, but I really didn't care. The situation had unraveled and no one seemed to be following a schedule at this point. There were rumors we were going to get paid only for regular work shifts, and that ticked everybody off. Here we were, sacrificing ourselves to work under those horrid conditions, and we might not even get fully compensated for our time.

While I was looking in my bag for a pair of socks, my dad woke up. At first he looked a little disoriented, like he didn't know we were still in Hell.

"You up?"

"Umm... yeah. What time is it?"

"After three o'clock, I guess." '

He sat up and put on his glasses. He was sitting there in just his boxer briefs looking exhausted. "You feelin' all right, Dad?"

"Fine. Just hot as heck."

"Does your back still itch, Dad?"

"Here and there, but not too bad. That cream worked pretty good."

"Good. Are you hungry or thirsty?"

"This is unbelievable!"

"What's unbelievable Son?"

"Oh ... nothing, Dad ... I was just thinking out loud."

At this time Dr. Marcus was waking up; he looked very pale and appeared as if he was going to throw up. "Doc, you all right?"

"I don't think so ... my kidneys ... my kidneys and bladder are really hurting. Walking and swimming in all that toxic water the past couple of days might have gotten me sick."

I tried to lighten the mood. "Is there anything I can do besides help you take a piss?"

With a forced smile, he replied, "Can you go get me some Bactrim DS please?" Bactrim is an antibiotic commonly used for many infections, usually kidney or urinary tract ones. "Sure, let me finish here and I'll go get you some."

My dad turned to look at the doctor and saw how bad he looked. "Son, that's fine. Go get those pills for the doctor."

Before I left, I introduced the doc and my dad. Dr. Marcus said, "You have a good son there. I don't know too many sons who would do what he's doing there."

Smiling, my dad said, "Yeah. I'm pretty lucky to have a son like him."

After wiping the excess cream off of my hands, I went over to the clinic. At some time during the day, they took all of the medications out of the carts and put them in garbage bags just like we did on the 10th floor. I asked one of the nurses who was sitting in there in the dark if she knew where the Bactrim was.

"Dr. Marcus needs some Bactrim. He thinks he might have a kidney infection or something."

"Look in that bag right there. There might be some in there."

After looking through the whole bag, I didn't find what I needed. It took me looking through two more bags before I finally found some.

It was about this time Captain Stanfield, a rank official from the Intake Processing Center, walked in. He looked awful. He said, "I need a tetanus shot or some antibiotics, because I feel like hell. I've been in the water and flat boat for over 40 hours straight."

The few nurses in the second-floor clinic shined their flashlights around and looked at each other in disbelief as he continued. "We've been out in the water saving people and bringing them to higher ground. I have little cuts all over my body, and that water is nasty!"

While he continued to tell us about the horrors he had seen in The last day and a half, a nurse and a doctor came to look at Stanfield.

The doctor said it was all right to give him a tetanus shot and told one of the nurses to give him some Keflex (an antibiotic) four times a day for seven days. After a few more minutes of listening to what was going on out there, I decided to go back over by Dr. Marcus. He was lying on his back in obvious pain.

"Here you go, Doc. Do you need something to drink?"

"Yes, please, please if you have anything."

"I have some room-temperature water if you want it," I said.

"That'll work."

"All right, guys, I'm heading up to 10, see you later," I said. I started on my way to the 10th floor. I almost got to the stairwell, and I realized I forgot to tell my dad we might be leaving sometime that evening or the next morning. He appeared to be somewhat relieved when I told him.

The 10th floor was busy. There were two inmates sitting on the bench having their vital signs taken and another one in the medical office having stitches removed. I got a report from the day nurse; there wasn't much out of the ordinary going on. She told me to expect the inmates to be complaining a bit that evening, because all they got to eat that day was one sandwich and no water.

I decided to walk the tier on the north side, which turned out to be a mistake. As soon as I went down there, the inmates started bombarding me.

"This is bullshit!"

"We need something to drink! Where's our food? We're starving in here!"

"What y'all tryin' to do to us, kill us?"

"Our toilets don't work! This is nasty up in here!"

I could feel myself getting really tensed up so, I got everyone's attention. "Listen up! Hey, listen up! We're doing the best we can under the circumstances. The city is real fucked up! They have dead bodies floating all over the city! People are stranded on rooftops and attics out there. People are getting shot, raped, and attacked! You name it, it's happening. Half the city is on fire! I know this sucks, but it sucks for all of us! We're short on food just like y'all."

At this point, a couple of jerks blurted out, "Y'all probably holdin' the food for yourselves!"

"Y' all don't give a shit about us!"

I was really getting angry by then, "Y'all can believe what the hell you want to believe! I'm just tellin' you the way it is! The military looks like its takin' over the city. I would think they are goin' to get us supplies when they can." I was saying this, but I really wasn't sure. I stood there for a few minutes looking, listening, and answering as many questions as I could. I could see some of those guys were really scared. "Man, I need to speak to my people."

"Where them levees broke at? My grandma lives over by one of them levees."

Other inmates continued to bitch and complain, and nothing I said made any difference. I saw Nurse Favis out of the corner of my eye, so I just walked away from the tier and blocked out all of the yelling and screaming.

Favis was in the medical office pressing all kinds of buttons on her phone. I watched her do this for a couple of minutes.

"Who are you trying to call?" I asked.

Laughing a little, she said, "I'm trying to use my text messaging on my phone to send a message to my mom, but it's not going through. Somebody downstairs was able to use theirs earlier on the roof." I grabbed my pockets for my phone, but realized it was downstairs in my bag. I asked, "I wonder if I can do that on my phone. I haven't tried it yet."

After making the rounds on the tiers and getting the same response from just about everybody, I went downstairs to get my phone. I hadn't eaten all day and was pretty hungry. The good side to that was I didn't use the bathroom, which made it worth it.

It was around 5 p.m. by the time I got to my bag. My dad was eating raviolis out of a can. When I saw that, my hunger level went down a notch. "I can't see how you could eat that without heating it up. That looks gross."

Looking at me, he said, "It's so damn hot in here already, you don't need to heat anything up." He had a point there. Just about everyone was down to shorts and a T-shirt.

Some people were down to their underwear, which was a little disgusting.

I could hear the sounds of babies crying in the distance. With the sun beating down on the building all day, staying inside was just about intolerable. The second floor was like a big kiln. No air was circulating at all. Even though we were near one of the only windows, it didn't help. I'm sure at some point there were people suffering from heat exhaustion, and I wasn't going to be surprised if we had a death or two from the heat before it was all over.

I grabbed my cell phone and told my dad I was heading back upstairs. With his mouth full of raviolis, he nodded and waved bye to me. Making that trip up the stairs was getting harder and harder.

Going off pure adrenaline by then, I felt like I was going to pass out when I got to the 10th floor. After each trip, it took longer to catch my breath. After a few minutes of deep breathing, I turned my phone on. Still no signal or indication that it was going to work. I asked Favis if she had had any luck, and she said he hadn't.

I went into the area where the St. Bernard deputies were so I could listen to the radio. The mood was still somber, obviously, but there were periods of anger voiced by several local political officials throughout the broadcast.

While listening to the radio, I heard the police chief of Kenner (where I live), describing the aftermath of the storm. "I'm riding down Williams Boulevard, and the water is anywhere from three to six feet high. We're turning west on Vintage Drive, and the water level appeared to be six feet at one time, based on the water line on the buildings ..." Of all the streets he could have been on he was about two to three blocks from my condo! I now had confirmation that my home was flooded along with my car.

The situation was getting grimmer by the hour. I began to wonder what my dad's place was like. I knew his car was swamped. If his home was too, this was going to be a complete disaster. If my Aunt Gladys' house was flooded, we wouldn't have any other place to stay in the metropolitan area. I had no idea where we would live or where my dad would live.

As I was contemplating this, a message popped up on my phone. I heard a beep, and it vibrated a little bit; the only time it usually does that is when I have my phone on silent and I get a phone call. I saw I had a text message. I had never used text messaging before, so said to Favis, "Hey, look at this. Please show me how to get the message."

She took the phone and pressed a couple of buttons and showed me the screen. It said, "R U OK. WE MISS U AND LOVE U. LORA AND FAMILY." I immediately felt a surge of energy.

"Look at that, Favis. How do I respond back?"

She showed me and told me when you send a message, a confirmation statement pops up on the screen when it goes through.

I tried to message my wife's phone, but the screen said, "Message failed." I tried again with the same results.

"Hey, Favis, why is this not working?"

"Sometimes the signal may not be strong enough or the number you're messaging isn't in a place where it can receive it."

"Great. That figures," I replied.

"Is your phone working?"

"No G; I'm gonna try tomorrow if we're still here.

Hopefully, we'll be outta here!"

"I hope so, but they haven't even moved any of the inmates in here yet." She looked at me with a shrug and a forced smile and said, "Oh well."

We sat there in silence for a few minutes. I could hear the occasional inmate asking for this or that and the radio announcer talking about the devastation in and around the city. I decided to go down to the roof of the mezzanine level to see if my text messaging would work.

The sun was setting, and the moon was visible in the distance. Some stars started to gleam and twinkle. The black smoke from the explosion still flowed in the sky. The other fires visible from the mezzanine roof still burned. There were fewer military helicopters than earlier in the day, but I could still hear them flying around.

There were empty bottles of water on the roof scattered in an area near the entrance. I walked to the far left-hand part of the roof to see if I could get a signal. I tried my wife's number, but it didn't work. I decided to scroll through my phone list to get my sister-in-law and brother -in-law's phone numbers to see if they would work. On my second try, I got Brian's (my brother-in-law) number to work and I sent a message. It read, "IM OK. DAD OK 4 NOW. VERY HOT AND MISERABLE. LOVE U, GAVIN."

After three tries, I finally got a confirmation message. At that point, I assumed my family got the message. As I went to go back inside, I saw Robert, and he said, "Be ready to go in the morning! You can only bring one bag, and they may not let you bring anything. Pack one bag just in case they let you take one."

Feeling positive for the first time in awhile, I replied, "Thanks! We'll be ready."

I decided to go down and tell my dad the good news. When I got down there, the diesel smell had taken over the second floor. It was dark but tubes of light from flashlights shined around like lasers. The news of our possible departure in the morning had everyone talking. When I got to my dad, he was smiling. "I guess you heard we might be leaving in the morning?"

"Finally. This heat is killing me!"

"Have you been drinking some water, Dad?"

"Yeah, but I could sure go for a cup of coffee."

"Hopefully wherever they bring us, we can get you some coffee."

"Do you need anything?"

"No, Son. I'm all right. I hope I can get my medicine tomorrow wherever we go."

"That would be nice, Dad, but I wouldn't count on it."

After about a minute or so, it dawned on me I had to decide what to take and what to leave behind. Looking at my dad through the candlelight I said, "Hey, we can only take one bag each, so I'm going to stuff as much as I can in my blue duffel bag and you can put what you want in my black duffel bag. We'll just leave your old suitcase behind." It was old as dirt anyway.

With a mildly disappointed look on his face, he replied,

"I guess so. Whatever we have to do to get the hell out of here, I'll do it! Hell, I'll walk out of here with no clothes on if I have to."

Laughing and getting a quick (bad) visual image, I mockingly said, "That won't be necessary, but thanks for letting me know that."

I started to rearrange what I thought we would need, changing my mind a couple of times. I had my father-in-law Gary's movies, about 20 or so, and my portable DVD player and was torn whether to take them or leave them behind. After a couple of minutes, I decided to just pack them in the bag as tightly as I could.

I took my other duffel bag and put my dad's stuff and the rest of my things in there. While I was packing, I heard on the radio people, I assumed looters or gangs, were shooting at military helicopters trying to land on top of hospitals, mainly Charity. I couldn't believe what I was hearing! It was odd. Here I am in a jail, and I feel safer than if I were out in the open somewhere in the city.

With all the lawlessness and turmoil, at least our criminals were behind bars ... for now.

After picking up each bag, I was hoping I wouldn't have to walk too far because they were quite heavy. I decided to leave my pillow (of course my favorite pillow) and the air mattresses behind, plus a few pieces of clothing. I thought I'd better go back up to the 10th floor to see if anything was going on. Since the first night, things had been crazy at times and relatively quiet at times, thank God. We obviously didn't have the capabilities to treat a life-or-death situation, and the facility was unable to access local hospitals.

Just before I went upstairs, I saw Nurse Urban's mother entering the bathroom with a box of gloves and cleaning supplies in her hands. I couldn't believe my eyes. She was actually going to clean that toxic cesspool of a bathroom. Anybody who would voluntarily do that deserves a Medal of Honor. I offered her the choice of anything I had to eat, "When you're done just look in this orange bag here. Take whatever you want."

With her Latin accent, she said, "Oh, tank you berry mooch. You berry kind."

I told my dad, "She's cleaning the bathroom; let her have anything she wants to eat."

"She's cleaning that bathroom?! Hell. She can have all of it if she wants. Wow!" My dad and I both looked at each other and shook our heads. I don't know how long it took her to do it and I almost gag every time I think of her cleaning that filth! I told my dad I was going back upstairs for a while and I would see him later. I stopped on the mezzanine level to look outside.

Walking out on the roof was like stepping into a whole new world: The night sky took my breath away. For a second straight night, the sky was completely illuminated with stars. It looked like there were more stars in the sky than darkness. It felt so surreal, as if I were in outer space. Standing there looking straight up, I again had that strange, spiritual feeling of a higher power controlling all of it. New Orleans had been so screwed up for so long, maybe divine intervention was the only way it was going to get fixed. With all of the corrupt politicians, judges, and criminals, maybe this event might be what was needed to get things turned around.

A cleansing?

It's a shame, because a lot of good people were suffering, but maybe it would get all the crooks to keep their hands out of the cookie jar. I could only hope. There are many good things about New Orleans, but the bad sometimes outweighs the good.

I stood there a little longer thinking. It was all happening so fast, yet being there, everything was in slow motion. A few seconds later I heard the crackle of gunfire in the distance. I instinctively ducked down and covered my head; maybe this roof wasn't the best place to be at night.

Turning to go back upstairs, I ran into Deputy Rico. He was with his family. Believe it or not, with the moonlight and the brightness of the stars, it was possible to make out figures and see a little bit.

"Hey, Gavin ... come meet my family."

Deputy Rico recently moved to New Orleans from California and was new to the hurricane experience. He sure picked a heck of a hurricane start with. Anyhow, he made a decision earlier in the day to bring his family on the roof and let them sleep out there for the night. It was kind of like camping without the trees and wildlife, unless you consider what was going on in the city as wildlife. "Gavin, this is my wife ... my daughter ... my son ... and my ..." All in all, he had about seven or eight people with him, and they were all set up on the roof with sleeping bags and pillows.

"You got 'em all set real good up here."

"Yeah, it sure beats the inside. It's getting miserable in there!"

I said, "Getting miserable? It's downright pitiful! You see the bathroom lately?"

"Unfortunately, I have, and it's unbelievable."

"Urban's mom had started to clean it up when I was on my way up here."

His jaw nearly hit the ground.

"You're kidding. That's unreal."

"I wouldn't have believed it if I didn't see it with my own eyes." After a few more minutes of small talk, I told him I had to go back upstairs.

I thought about asking my dad if he wanted to come up to the roof, but then thought better of it. I had mental images of him wandering around in the middle of the night and falling off the side of the building into the water, never to be seen again.

When I got to the 10th floor, the inmates were chanting, ranting and raving. Favis was sitting in the office with the door closed. She just smiled and said, "They're getting louder and louder with that crap."

It was about 9:15 p.m. or so and I was about fed up with dealing with the inmates. I understood their frustration, but we were all in the same boat. No matter what we said they didn't believe us, so what was the use of trying to explain the situation anymore?

J.W. seemed to be doing all right — physically, but he really didn't comprehend what was going on.

I made the mistake of letting him see me, and he shouted, "Dad, when are we going home?"

I hesitated for a second or two before I answered, because I could see he was sincere.

"J.W. listen, we've had a real bad rainstorm and it's flooded outside. They're going to move us to somewhere where it's not flooded."

I could hear someone laughing because I was talking to him like a kid, but that was his state of mind. I turned to the guy who was laughing and said, "Will you shut the hell up, man?"

"Yeah man. I was just playin'," he replied.

"Not right now please. Thanks." J.W was waiting for me to continue. "Like I was saying J.W., we're going to be leaving soon. You're going to be all right."

He told me to come close to the cell so he could whisper.

"Are you coming with me?" Not wanting to upset him, I said, "Probably so ... go lie down and try to get some sleep, okay?"

"All right, Dad, see you later!"

I went back into the office for a little while and tried to use my text messaging with no success. I was listening to the radio, and I heard the announcer say, "The Gentilly and New Orleans East area is inundated with water. Anywhere from eight to ten feet of water covering the area ..."

My heart sank in my chest thinking of the fertility clinic where our embryos were frozen in New Orleans East. There was a real possibility everything was now flooded, maybe even destroyed. I just put my head down and prayed everything would be all right. Along with everything else potentially lost, this would be the hardest to deal with.

"Hey Favis, I'm heading downstairs. I've had enough for today. I'll see if Urban will come up early."

"Okay, G, that's cool. See ya later." I went back downstairs to the second floor. When I got to our spot, it was very dark with the only light coming from a candle on the table. It was the same candle with the image of Jesus on it.

Dr. Marcus, Urban, his mother, my dad, and Dr. Singh were sitting and lying around. Urban saw me and said, "Aren't you supposed to be up on 10 right now?"

"Yeah, but I had enough of that today; besides Favis is up there and it's fairly quiet, except for the complaining and occasional chanting."

Looking concerned, Urban said, "Does she need any help?"

"I told her I'd see if you would want to go up there early. Would you?"

He looked at his watch and said, "It's only ten after ten. I'll go up in about half an hour."

I changed my shirt and sprayed on some deodorant; I was sure I smelled pretty bad. I tried my deflated mattress and shot back in frustration. "I just bought this stupid air mattress, and it ain't worth damn!" I lifted up my mattress and used Urban's flashlight to see why it was deflated. Everything looked good until I spotted a little sliver of glass from the shattered window. I couldn't see a hole in the mattress, but it most likely came from broken glass.

That figures. I guess I'll just lay out some clothes and sleep on them!

Once I got settled in, we all started talking. I don't remember how we got on the subject, but we started talking about where the inmates were going. Someone said, "That's gonna' be screwed up if someone is in here on a drunk in public charge and now they'll be somebody's "girlfriend" up at Angola." We all burst out laughing.

Dr. Marcus chimed in next, "So if somebody was arrested for a traffic violation, they're going to end up at Angola Penitentiary?"

"Possibly," I said. "I know we have a couple people who were scheduled to roll out Monday. They'll end up at Angola too."

Dr. Singh just looked at us under the soft candlelight with a smirking smile and said, "You guys are terrible." She was right. But it was sort of humorous — so long as it wasn't us. We continued entertaining ourselves with different scenarios that might play out for the unlucky souls who were leaving our facility.

Then Dr. Marcus brought us up to date on the evacuation of the Medical Observation Unit and told us how some of the medical staff couldn't swim, so they had to use garbage cans and benches to float the medical staff to the CCC building. As the conversation slowed down, Urban left to go up to the 10th floor, and I could see that my dad was starting to dose off.

"Hey, Dad, good night. Love you, Buddy."

"Good night, Son. Love you." Soon he was asleep.

Chapter 14

Hope

Even though our building wasn't evacuated yet, I was feeling pretty confident we would be leaving the next day. Trying to cool down, I took my sweaty shirt off. Even at 11 p.m., everybody was sweating profusely, and the only way to generate any breeze was to fan myself with something. I grabbed the pillow in the middle and started fanning my dad again.

I found myself staring at the candle on the table. The way it was flickering it seemed to project the Jesus-like image on the wall. The candle had some Spanish writing on it, and I'm not sure if it was Jesus or not. Still, it was oddly comforting.

I felt myself smiling at the candle, and every time I did, it seemed like the flame got brighter and the image on the wall got bigger. I don't know if I was hallucinating from the heat, but when I wasn't smiling the flame didn't appear as bright or the image as big. It changed when I smiled or looked at it and it always got brighter and bigger. I did this for a while, becoming somewhat mesmerized by this mystical occurrence. Peculiar, I know.

Just about everyone was sleeping. I noticed the smell from the bathroom wasn't as bad as before. Nurse Urban's mother must have really done a great job. God bless her!

For the next hour or so, I continued fanning my dad and trying to block out the sound of occasional gunshots in the distance. The way things had gone so far, I was hoping no stray bullets would find their way through our windows. By this time, I was thinking of all kinds of crazy scenarios. I decided to eat a granola bar since I hadn't had anything to eat all day. While munching on it and drinking room temperature, in this case hot, water, I caught myself looking at the candle again and again. The flame would get brighter and brighter. I got chills on my neck, and a calming feeling came over me. It seemed otherworldly. I truly felt a supernatural presence. After a while, I turned over to try and get some sleep on my bed of lumpy clothes.

I don't know what time it was in the morning, but it was still dark. I was half asleep when I felt someone shaking my left arm and whispering my name, "Gavin ... Son, wake up." I sat up, one of my clammy shirts stuck to my face. I was covered with sweat and the stench from the bathroom was back. "Son, I gotta go to the bathroom."

Trying to get my bearings I said something like, "Let me grab the flashlight, and I'll go with you."

I tore off part of the remaining piece of sheet, grabbed a roll of toilet paper and told my dad to hold on to my shoulder and follow the light. He fumbled with his eyeglasses a bit, but got them on. I had to hold in a laugh because when he stood up, his hair was standing straight up on the left side of his head and all he had on was his boxer shorts and a pair of my flip-flops, which were a little too small.

We tip-toed our way to the bathroom and when we got in there, I saw this five gallon bucket with a rope tied to the handle and the other end of the rope tied to a leg of the counter where the sinks were. I went over to the toilets and saw the bad news. It hadn't taken long for the bathroom to get back to its horrible state. It was amazing to me so many people had such little respect for the facility and everyone else there. I looked up and saw a sign on the door that said,

"NO PAPER IN THE TOILET!" I said to myself, No paper in the toilet ... that's all they had in the toilets in addition to you know what."

Then my dad said, "What are you doing, Son?"

"I'm trying to figure out what to do ... you can't go in either one of these."

I looked at the bucket and looked at the sheet in my hand and said, "Here's your toilet right here." I took the sheet and tore enough to line the bucket. "All right, Dad, have a seat."

Looking tentative, he said, "I don't know, Son. I don't know if I can go in that."

"Well, that's your only choice right now, everything else is too nasty and you could get sick. So give it a try." I helped him get positioned on the bucket and stepped over by the door to give him his privacy.

After he finished, he said, "Well, Son, I've never done that before." We laughed and took the sheet and wrapped the little present up and threw it out the window. The way I saw it, we really didn't have a choice. We went back to our spot and my dad laid back down. I grabbed my pillow and fanned him until he fell back asleep. I didn't get to see what time it was, but it was still dark outside. Before I knew it, I was asleep.

I awoke to loud voices outside the window; I could hear boat motors going and what sounded like people giving commands.

"DON'T MOVE! DO AS WE SAY!"

"KEEP YOUR HANDS WHERE WE CAN SEE THEM!"

I looked out the window, and every few minutes I saw a small flat boat go by with inmates in the middle and armed guards sitting on the edges. I decided to go up to the mezzanine to take a closer look.

When I got up there, I saw Nurse Robert and asked him if we were getting ready to leave. "Not yet. It may not even be today. I really don't know."

Deflated, I said, "You're kidding, right?"

"Nope. It's taking along time to move the inmates by boat. We can only get six to eight per boat and you know we got somethin' like six thousand to seven thousand inmates to move."

With my tone changing to exasperation I said, "Damn! I was sure we were leaving today."

I guess he could see I was frustrated, "Hang in there G. How's your dad?"

"Okay right now, but he thought we were leaving today. Plus, he's just about out of his medicine."

Looking like he really didn't know what to say, he replied, "I don't know what to tell you, dude. We're doin' the best we can."

"Oh, I know. Don't worry about it. I'll talk to you later."

Robert walked away, repositioning his rifle and scratching his backside in the same motion. I walked over by the south side of the roof and I could see inmates in boats. The Templeman buildings had inmates waving white sheets or towels out of the shattered, steel-barred windows and some other inmates sat on the roof with nowhere to go. I looked to my far right, and the CCC building had a window about six stories up with about five or six sheets or blankets tied together hanging out of it. I then looked to my far left toward the Broad Street Bridge, which was about 200 yards away; rows and rows of shackled inmates sat or squatted on the bridge, surrounded by men with guns. I then looked to the right of the inmates on the bridge and down below, I could see all types of buses on the I-10 Interstate taking inmates and civilians away. There was some type of ladder or slide set up from the bridge down to the highway below. People got off the boats and walked through the water below the bridge. In the distance, I could hear the loud roar of airboats sounding like racecars revving their engines. The sky was full of military and Red Cross helicopters. The scene was very apocalyptic.

I walked around the entire roof, taking it all in. I looked at my car one more time, and all I could see was about a foot of the top of it. My dad's car was completely submerged. The water was still rising with no apparent end in sight.

We were at one of the lowest spots in the city and I was at one of the lowest points in my life. It was at that moment I felt as if my dad and I were in Alcatraz Prison surrounded by toxic water, hoping we wouldn't have to swim to FREEDOM! I began to reflect on anything I might have done in my life that would have landed me in this situation. Was this situation a punishment for my younger, wilder days? I didn't know.

But what did my dad ever do to deserve this at 83? Some things just don't make sense.

I heard the loud roar of a military helicopter and when I was able to see it, I saw the helicopter drop some boxes of MREs, meals ready to eat, and more water. I had mixed feelings at this point, because I was grateful we were getting more supplies, but worried we may not be leaving anytime soon.

After the drop was completed, the people in charge started to organize and hand out supplies. I waited for a little while before I went over to see what they had. They asked, "How many people do you have with you?"

I answered, "My dad and I." I was given two brown plastic bags that were tightly sealed and hard like a box was in the bag. I also got two bottles of water. I took my supplies and went downstairs to see my dad.

When I got to our spot, he wasn't there. I opened one of the MREs to see what was inside. To my surprise, the food looked pretty good: a bag of M&Ms, peanuts, crackers, trail mix, and a main course of lasagna. I looked at it for a moment wondering how good lasagna would be out of a box. I was pretty hungry because I really had not eaten anything except a couple of granola bars the past couple of days. I decided to eat some of the trail mix and save the M&Ms for my dad, since he loves his chocolate.

A few minutes later, he walked up and said he was out of cigarettes. Half jokingly, I said, "Good." He didn't seem amused.

"Don't worry, Dad, give your lungs a break. I'll find you some later."

With an agitated look on his face he said, "Yeah, yeah, whatever," and I left it at that. I decided change the subject a bit and show him the MREs and give him the pack of M&Ms before I told him we were probably not going to leave that day.

While he was eating his M&Ms, I said casually, "It doesn't look like we'll be leavin' today."

He looked at me with total disappointment, "What? You are joking, right?"

Looking down, not wanting to make eye contact with him, I said, "Nope, they're still evacuating the other buildings and since only the first floor of our building is flooded and not up here yet, we'll probably be the last building evacuated."

Disgusted and upset he said, "Damn, Son! I guess I won't get my medicine any time soon." He had anxiousness on his face, and I knew there was nothing I could do about it.

"Listen, Dad — we have a couple of doctors here in case you have any problems."

"Yeah, but my meds!"

"I know ... I know. I already talked to one of the doctors and if you start having any trouble, I'm sure that we can give you some other comparable medication."

"I don't know about that, Son."

Trying not to sound perturbed, I replied, "Well, Dad, we really don't have a choice right now, unless you want to swim out of here."

"Could we do that?"

"Are you freakin' kiddin'? Even if we could, all the drug stores are getting looted, you know, broken into, or are on fire!"

Half slapping his leg, he blurted out, "Goddamn! What have I gotten myself into?"

At this point, I didn't say anything. I sat there on the floor and looked out of the nearby shattered window. My dad huffed and puffed for a couple of minutes and finished eating his M&Ms.

"Dad, I'll be back in a little while. As soon as I find out anything I'll let you know. Try and relax."

"Yeah, yeah," he said. And off I went.

It was mid-afternoon, I guess about 2 or 2:30, and I decided to go back to the roof. Once again, it was an extremely hot and muggy summer day without a cloud in the sky. There were plenty people on the roof now, and some of the deputies guarded a doorway that led to a parking garage next to our building. I found out it was a parking garage for the NOPD and some other vehicles like boats and motorcycles. They were using those vehicles to siphon off gas in order to keep the boats running. I also heard that batteries were being taken for power as well.

Who would have known we had our own looting going on?

The boats, obviously, were the only means of transportation, especially to move the inmates to the nearby bridge for evacuation.

When I was on the roof, Urban's mom, the lady who cleaned the foul bathroom, asked me to help her move some cardboard boxes in to the doorway to the roof because she said there was "aceed" (acid) leaking from the containers in the mezzanine area.

I asked her how she knew this and in her strong Spanish accent she said, "Me feet is a burning! Me shoes have been wet and they burning. Help me please cover the floor so no one else feet is burning!" She looked pretty adamant about doing this so we went back down to the second floor and started gathering up old cardboard boxes and anything we could use to cover the floor.

There were some blue tarps near the old cafeteria area and used cardboard boxes in the back of the second-floor medical clinic. Since there wasn't much light in the building, we had to drag the stuff around in the dark. We both tripped a couple times, but, luckily, weren't injured.

Once we finally got to the mezzanine area, we started to tear the cardboard boxes long-ways so they could cover more of the floor. There was about an inch or so of water and "acid" on the floor between the bottom of the metal stairs to the doorway. After laying down as many boxes as we could, we laid the tarp down and it covered almost to the doorway to the roof.

I thought we were finished, but she said, "Need more! Not enough. We find more." She was small in stature, but had this forceful demeanor about her.

Feeling like I didn't have much of a choice and trying to sound enthused, I said, "All right, let's go."

For the next half-hour or so, we searched the entire second floor for things we could use to cover the walkway. Many people sitting around were looking at us like we were nuts. I let her take the lead and didn't say much. When anyone gave me a strange look, I just shrugged my shoulders and grabbed what I could.

When we finally finished gathering and laying down what we could, it looked like someone had cut open a gigantic trash bag and poured it out in a straight line. It wasn't pretty, but it did the job. Luckily, I had thick shoes on, so I didn't know what she was feeling on her feet, but I could tell she was having some pain or burning sensation. I gave her a pair of my socks when we were done, and she cleaned her feet with a bottle of water and an old shirt. I'm not sure how many pairs of feet we saved from the "acid" and not many people knew why those boxes, tarps, and other stuff were on the floor, but at least we tried to solve the problem.

It was about mid-afternoon by then, and the heat was wicked. With a minimal breeze up on the roof, it had to be near 100 degrees with 98 percent humidity. After taking a 15minute break, I went to go check on my dad. He was facing the wall, wearing only his boxer shorts. I thought he was asleep, but he surprised me by calling my name.

"Oh, hey, Dad. I thought you were sleeping."

"It's too damn hot, and my back is itching like crazy. My lower back is hurting as well."

"Hang on a second, and I'll rub some of that anti-itch cream on your back." I sat down for a second and drank some warm water and dug around to find the cream.

I was in the middle of putting the cream on his back when Dr. Marcus, Nurse Technician Michelle and a couple of the nurses rushed to our area near the window by the incoming light. I turned to see what all the commotion was, and I saw Michelle holding her right index finger with a bloody shirt wrapped around it. Michelle was just about to take her test to be a licensed nurse before the storm and was well on her way to being a great nurse. At some point between Wednesday night and the time she showed up right behind me, they broke out all of the small windows on the 10th floor to help with air circulation. She was up on the ledge looking out the window on the 10th floor and when she jumped down, her hand was on the window and her right index finger snagged a piece of the jagged glass and cut it down to the bone. Her makeshift bandage was completely soaked with blood.

She must have cut an artery because blood was squirting out every other second when Dr. Marcus uncovered it. Her finger looked like a shrimp that had been "butterflied" open, and blood squirted with every heartbeat. The nurses came back with sutures and supplies to stitch up her finger. The cut was so deep Dr. Marcus was concerned about the tendons being permanently damaged and infection setting in. I hurriedly wiped my hands off and told my dad to wait a minute so I could help.

We set up a sterile field (as sterile as we could get the area), and the doc deadened the cut with Lidocaine and began to clean the wound with Betadine antiseptic. He carefully began stitching up the wound. There were a few people standing around watching intently. Michelle couldn't bear to watch.

We were joking with each other, and I tried to loosen her up with some jokes. "Nice trigger finger. At least you've got four good ones left!" It seemed to calm her down by the few forced laughs she let out.

It took Dr. Marcus 30 minutes or so to close the wound. He asked Nurse Favis to go get her some Keflex (antibiotic) to take in case any infection set in. Dr. Marcus was totally exhausted by this point and was quite proud of his work. "I have to say that was one of the toughest stitch jobs I've ever done. With the cut down to the bone, she really needed surgery, but I think I got it done!"

After patting himself on the back for a second, he got serious and said, "I have to warn you that your finger may not come back 100 percent the way it was before, and the risk of infection is quite high."

I could see the concern on her face as she sarcastically replied, "That's great."

Dr. Marcus continued with, "Keep it bandaged up for a couple of days and when you change it, make sure your hands are clean."

She nervously asked, "I'm not going to lose my finger, am I?"

"No, no. Keep taking the antibiotics and keep it clean, and you should be okay."

She didn't look convinced and yelled, "I can't believe this shit!"

Before Favis and another nurse bandaged the finger, I took one last look at it. I think he used 12 to 15 stitches and the wound looked like a small zipper on her finger. While the other nurses covered the wound, she asked me if I had spoken to the rest of my family lately. "Not since Monday night. I got a text message yesterday and sent one back, but I don't know if they got it."

She looked at me and said, "They have some deputies on the 10th floor who are able to call and get calls."

I looked at her with amazement and asked, "What? How?"

Dr. Marcus heard what she said and said something to the same effect.

At about that moment, Dr. Marcus and I stood up and Urban walked up to see what was going on. I went over to my bag to grab some water and said, "I'm going to 10 to see if I can get a hold of Lora!"

Dr. Marcus and Urban simultaneously said, "We're coming too!"

Dr. Marcus then said, "Gavin, can I use your phone when we get up there?"

"Hell yeah, Doc. Lets go!"

When we got to the 10th floor, I saw about 15 deputies with phones in their hands trying to make calls. Deputy Avery was sitting with his head down and his hands on top of his head, looking distraught. "What's up Avery? You all right?"

"No man. I don't know what's up with my girl and my 8- month-old baby boy. The last time I heard their voices was on the radio, and she was calling from the attic of our place."

I didn't quite know what to say. I couldn't imagine a worse scenario for his family. "Where do you live?"

"In the East (New Orleans East), man. In the East." I stood there looking out of the window, feeling awfully bad for him.

I waited a couple of seconds before saying, "Man, stay positive. At least her voice went out over the radio. Hopefully, they got help."

"Yeah, thanks G." But I wasn't so sure he was convinced.

I waited for a couple of minutes before trying to use my phone.

Everyone was dialing and trying to speak quickly because the signals were fading in and out. One of the female deputies said, "Stand over to your right by the corner and squat down a little bit. You might get a signal."

I tried that a couple of times with no luck.

Dr. Marcus asked me if he could try my phone. I took a step back and let him get near the corner where I was. He tried for a few minutes with no luck either. Urban had his phone with him and gave it to Dr. Marcus as well. Still no luck.

It's amazing we can build a space station and go to the moon, but we can't keep telephones working here on earth!

Another female deputy offered me her phone. "Hey G, try my phone, but only for a couple of minutes."

"Hey thanks." I tried Lora's cell phone number and on third or fourth ring, she answered, "Hello? Gavin! Gavin!"

"Hey baby, it's me!"

She immediately started crying saying, "Are you all right?

They have ... all kinds of crazy stuff on CNN! Like ..." "Hey, hey, calm down. I'm all right. What are they saying?"

"They're saying that ... that ... there's a riot at the prison. That they have hostages. That there are people — getting shot!"

Trying to reassure her, I said, "Nothing has happened in this building, yet. It's just miserably hot, and we're surrounded by water. I don't know when we're going to be evacuated. Just know I'm barely making it for now."

She started to cry more, barely catching her breath. "How's your Dad?"

"He's alive. I think he's just hanging in there."

"What do you mean?" Realizing I was not using my phone and other people needed to use it I said, "Nothing ... hey, listen, I'm using someone else's phone. I think this text messaging thing works on my phone — I got a text yesterday from ya'll ... did you get mine?"

"No, no ... you're breakin' up a little."

"I'm okay right now. I'll try to call you later. Love you."

"What. .. I can't hear you"

"I love you! I'll call you later."

I faintly heard her say, "I love you too," and the call was dead.

At that moment I let out a sigh of relief, but then realized neither of us was sure what was going on. All I knew was our building was secure at that time. Dr. Marcus and Urban were waiting rather impatiently for the phone. I went to hand the phone back to the female deputy and she must have seen the looks on their faces, because she said, "Give it to the Doc!"

I turned back around toward Dr. Marcus and she said over my shoulder, "Two minutes, Doc, and you too."

"Oh, Jesus. Thanks."

For the next few minutes both the doctor and nurse tried to call whoever it was they were trying to call, with no success. I stood there with all kinds of emotions going on. I looked to my left and saw Deputy Avery just looking down with a blank stare on his face.

Another deputy was talking adamantly with a family member about something, another deputy was on her phone laughing about something, and to my right Dr. Marcus was frantically dialing numbers with no success. Urban was dialing his phone with no success either, but I had been able to at least hear Lora's voice, and she at least knew my dad and I were all right and not hostages.

At least not yet.

I turned to Urban and said, "You're not gonna believe what they're saying on national news. That the jail has been taken over and that there are hostages and riots! Stuff like that!"

With his mouth opening wide he said, "You kidding?"

"That's what she said. Is that freakin' crazy or what? I wonder if something happened in one of the other buildings and they're just not saying anything?"

"Who knows? All I know is I don't think we're leavin' anytime soon."

"I hope you're wrong, but you're probably right."

Just as I was saying that, my phone vibrated in my pocket. I grabbed it and looked at the screen and it read, "WE ALL LUV U AND MISS U; BE SAFE. CALL ME WHEN U CAN. I LUV U VERY MUCH. LORA."

I felt so helpless. I stared at the screen for a minute, contemplating when we might get out of there. It was noisy, with everyone talking to each other or on the phone. I took my phone and asked one of the female deputies to make sure I was sending my response text correctly.

"Do this, and press that and that should be it."

I sent back a text saying, "LUV U 2. IM OK. HOPE TO SEE U SOON. GAVIN."

After I sent the message, I got the confirmation "message sent" about 15 seconds later. Dr. Marcus was standing there looking frustrated and Urban looked just plain angry. "Doc, who are you trying to call?"

"Mainly my daughter. She lives in Baton Rouge."

"You wanna try my phone again? You could try to text message her."

"What's that?"

"Here, I'll show you. Give me the number you're trying to call."

For the next couple minutes, we tried to send text messages for Dr. Marcus and Urban, but unfortunately, neither one went through. I happened to look up at one of the broken windows and saw what looked like a little bloodstain on one of the jagged pieces of glass.

"Hey, were any of you up here when Michelle cut her finger?" I asked.

A couple deputies said "Yeah," and one pointed to the spot I was looking at and said, "She was leaning against the window right there and I don't know what happened, but the next thing I know she was holding her finger and blood was all over her hand."

A couple of other deputies echoed the story, saying blood was everywhere. There were some dried droplets on the floor and on the ledge. I know for a fact those windows are not cleaned very often and are probably filled with all kinds of germs. I hoped nothing bad would happen to Michelle, since there wasn't much we could do if she got seriously ill.

It was after 3:30 p.m. and hot as Hades. I went to go to the back of the 10th floor to look in one of the storage areas to see if there was any Gatorade left. I was last in there on Tuesday and there was about a half a case at that time. When I got to the storage room, the pad lock was broken off and the door was slightly open. The room had been cleaned out. Looted, I guess. I went back over to the barred window area and saw a deputy.

"What happened to the storage door?"

"You know G; it's hot up here. We had to get our drink on!"

"I hear ya ... hey, have you talked to your wife at all?" I asked.

"No, man. I begged her to come here or evacuate, but she didn't want to. I don't know man. I'm tryin' not to think about it."

Remembering his family, I asked, "Don't you have kids?"

"Three, G. Three kids now. I'm prayin' they're gonna be all right."

I was really feeling fortunate. This was the second deputy I talked to who had no idea if his family was alive or dead.

"Hey, man, I hope everything will be all right."

"Me too, G. Me too."

Again, I thought of our embryos, what could potentially have been our children. New Orleans East was under water, and the fertility clinic probably was also. Our last in-vitro transfer could be affected. I could only hope the necessary precautions were taken in the event of an emergency. I lowered my head for a minute and prayed. It was so important to us. I wondered if Lora was thinking of them too.

I went over to an open space by the window and looked out toward the Broad Street Bridge in the middle of the city. I had to look twice at an area in front of where the inmates were. There were two inmates lying half on their side and face down. "Hey y'all, look at those inmates lying face down on the bridge. You think they have been shot or what?"

Just about everybody looked. One of the male deputies said, "He's been lyin' there for as long as I have been up here. At least two hours." I was trying to see any signs of blood, but it was too far away to tell.

It still looked like organized chaos on the bridge. There were civilians sitting and walking around on one side and hundreds of inmates either sitting or squatting in rows surrounded by some deputies with guns and other military personnel. Helicopters still flew all over the city. The water now covered most of the interstate up to the area under the bridge. Someone went to go get a radio, and as soon as it came on the announcer said, "There are reports of people trying to walk across the Crescent City Connection Bridge and being stopped by the Gretna police on the West Bank side of the bridge.

There were even reports of gunfire! I repeat: there are ..." Everybody kind of looked shocked.

Someone shouted, "This is unbelievable man!" We all got quiet and listened to the radio. I really don't remember what else was broadcast, but none of it was good.

After a while, I decided to go back downstairs to check on my dad. I didn't have my flashlight with me, so I just used the handrails and walked down in the dark. Believe it or not, as bright as it was outside, it was just as dark in the stairwell. I was going along, taking my time, but when I got to the sixth floor I started to hear a bunch of male voices barking out commands like, "Don't move! Do exactly as we say! Shut the fuck up! Don't move!"

As I made the turn on the stairwell right before the doorway to the fifth floor tier, I got the scare of a lifetime. When I stepped off of the last step there was a jet-black wolf-looking dog with piercing eyes and gnashing teeth looking right up at me. The only way I was able to see this vicious creature was from the sliver of light coming through the opening tier door.

Attached to a thick leash, it was held back by some sort of armed military-type man. There were quite a few of those men; I saw they had "DOC" (Department of Corrections) on their shirts and hats. I stopped dead in my tracks and backed up a few feet against the wall.

It took me a second or two to realize this creature was actually a German Sheppard. I had never seen a one like that. It looked like some sort of wolf dog, but more wolf. Its ravenblack coat was extremely shiny, and its eyes were bright yellow with beady pupils. While mesmerized by this animal, I could hear the cell gates opening and orders being yelled at the inmates.

After I stood still for about 10 seconds, the man holding the leash moved forward through the doorway. The dog looked me right in the eye for a second and then went through the door down the fifth floor tier.

Those inmates aren't going to like seeing that scary wolf-dog coming at them!

I couldn't help myself – I took a look down the tier and it was full with men toting sawed-off shotguns, a couple more police dogs, and inmates with their hands on their heads looking extremely scared. One last guy came through the doorway, kind of bumping me out of the way.

I decided to go downstairs before they accidentally lumped me in with the inmates or something. Stepping down the rest of the stairwell, I started having visions of those vicious black dogs tearing me to pieces. I was getting really unnerved.

When I got to the second floor, most everyone must have realized they were starting to evacuate the inmates. I overheard a group of people say, "We gotta' be gettin' outta' here soon!"

"Yeah, you right."

When I got to my dad, he was eating some crackers, sitting on his mattress looking bored out of his skull.

"Hey, Dad, they're starting to move the inmates out of this building."

"Oh, so we're leaving today?"

"That I don't know. You feelin' all right?"

"I'm getting a little dizzy every now and then. That's about all, other than the heat."

Grabbing my duffel bag and getting my blood pressure cuff and stethoscope, I said, "Sit back against the wall so I can check your blood pressure and pulse."

After positioning his sweaty arm, I placed the BP cuff and stethoscope in position and got a reading of 150/98. High, but not alarming. His pulse was strong and slightly rapid. I figured with the heat and his age, he was probably still a little dehydrated. For that matter, we were all probably dehydrated.

I decided to tell him it was a little lower than it was so he wouldn't worry. Looking at me, he said "Is it all right?"

"Yeah, Dad ... uh, it's not bad. How many pills do you have left?"

Troubled, he said, "One more day's worth."

"We'll be out of here soon."

Looking more disconcerted, he said, "You keep sayin' that, but we're still here!"

"I know, but they're moving the inmates as we speak. Hey, I almost forgot to tell you, I was able to talk to Lora for a couple of minutes upstairs."

"She's upstairs?"

Laughing, I said, "I was able to get in contact with her on the cell phone from the 10th floor. I was able to get some reception up there."

"Oh, is she all right?"

"Yeah. She's in Paris, Texas with family. That is where they evacuated."

"I wish I was in Texas right now."

"Me too, Dad. Me too."

We sat there in silence for a few minutes. I decided to go up to the mezzanine roof to see what was going on and to find out if we were leaving any time soon. "I'll be back in a minute, Dad."

I went to the roof with the intention of finding Robert to see if he had any new news. On my way there I saw somebody, I can't really remember who, but they said, "I heard we're going to be evacuated to the Convention Center and then onto a Coast Guard ship and brought to Houston."

With my heart sinking in my chest I said, "What? Where did you hear that?"

"One of the rank told me that."

This can't be happening! It's going to take us forever to get there from here, to the Convention Center, on a boat, and then to Houston by boat.

Dejected, I trudged back up to the stairs to the roof to find Deputy Robert. After walking the perimeter of the roof for a few minutes, I saw him standing over by the entry to the adjacent elevated parking lot, where they were siphoning the gas.

As I walked toward him, I saw an inmate jumping from an area down to the roof of the other building and then lying on his side, grabbing his leg. There was another inmate sitting near where this inmate jumped to. Were they making an escape? I wonder where they think they're going... surrounded by water and men with guns.

I made my way over to Robert, and asked him if there was any news. "Not really, Gav. The only thing I do know is that they plan on moving any sick or elderly people first, so your dad ..."

I shot back, "I can't be separated from him! I don't know how he's doing mentally and physically; he could be suffering from dehydration."

"No, no! You would be able to go with him."

"Do you know where?"

"Nope. I've heard all kinds of places — Convention Center, Houma (south Louisiana), Houston, San Antonio."

"Yeah, I heard maybe to the Convention Center, then to Houston on a Coast Guard boat."

"It's possible. Who knows?"

"As long as we get the hell outta' here!"

"I guess you're right. Thanks. I'll see you later."

"Later, Gavin."

I slowly walked over to an area of the roof where there weren't too many people. I stood there for a while, sweating profusely, watching the evacuation process unfold. I looked straight across from where I was standing and I couldn't believe my eyes. There was an elderly lady holding a poster board-sized sign against a tinted window that read, "HELP!"

I thought I was seeing things, so I rubbed my eyes and looked again. Sure enough "HELP!" was plastered to the window. I started to wave at the window for a few seconds when she finally put the sign down. I tried to yell to her, but she couldn't hear me. I made a signal so as to say, "Wait a second, I'll be right back," and ran back over to where Robert was, but he wasn't there. I asked one of the deputies, and he said he thought he went down to the second floor.

I went down there and after about five minutes of looking for him, I found him in one of his father-in-law's offices. "Hey Robert, there's an older woman on the top floor of the Municipal Court building holding a sign in the window that says, 'Help!'"

He stood up and said, "What? Where?"

I insisted, "Follow me, I think you can see her from the window over by my stuff."

We walked together and when we got there, sure enough, we could see her holding her sign.

"How long has she been there?" Robert asked.

"I have no idea," I told him. "I just saw her a few minutes ago when I was on the roof. Can you do anything for her?"

"I'm going to go find a radio and let someone know she's in there."

A few other people stood near us, looking at her. Periodically, she would put the sign down and wave to us again. As Robert walked off, a few of us made gestures to the lady; trying to encourage her. Since the window was solid and not broken that was all we could really do to communicate with her. It looked like she smiled and acknowledged us. I couldn't tell if she was by herself or not. We tried to get her to give us any indication if she was alone or not, but were unsuccessful in our attempts.

The few people standing around started to trickle off and, eventually, so did I. My dad was sitting down watching two little kids hitting each other, pushing each other, and just horsing around. "One of those kids is gonna get hurt," my dad told me.

Not even five seconds later one of the kids fell backward and hit his head against the metal cabinet. Of course, he started crying. Either the boy's mom or aunt, I guess, started hitting the other kid really hard and told him, "You stupid little #!*?" We sat there watching this unfold, and I really felt sorry for both of the kids.

My dad turned to me and whispered, "Damn, she's hitting the heck out of that kid'; she's gonna hurt him."

I shook my head in agreement and whispered back, "I'm glad you never did that to me; mom was a little rough with me, but not you."

"Well, Son, I never really believed in hitting a child."

"Yeah, Dad, I remember you shaking me when you were mad at me, but mom wouldn't hesitate to whack me a couple of times."

Half smiling at me he said, "You could be a handful when you were a kid, Son."

"Yeah, I probably did deserve a whack or two."

Shaking his head, my dad said, "Naw, Son, I learned a long time ago that spanking a child rarely did any good. Speaking of your mother, where is she anyway?"

"I honestly don't have a clue, Dad. I'm pretty sure she told me she was working on the train to Chicago. I think she told me she was leaving on Saturday or Sunday. I haven't spoken to her since last week some time."

"I hope she left the city."

"Me too, Dad. Me too."

We sat there for a few minutes watching the one kid crying and the other kid crying from the beating and scolding he took. The kid who had hit his head looked fine. It appeared he was crying more out of a need for attention than from pain.

The other boy was sitting by himself crying, looking at the woman every once in a while.

All of the sudden, my dad said, "You know you shouldn't hit that kid like that! You're gonna — "

The woman turned her head and yelled, "Don't tell me how to handle my child!"

Instantly, I felt like this might be trouble. My dad stammered, "Hold up lady ... I'm not telling you how to ..."

"Listen, mind your own business old man!"

At this point I stood up, holding my hand up and pointing at my dad to be quiet. I said, "Hey, hey, he didn't mean any harm lady. We're sorry." She kind of gave a defiant look and turned back to talk to her sister or cousin or whomever she was talking to before the little kid took his beating.

That's part of the problem with some kids and parents in New Orleans — they've lost their way. No one can tell anyone anything without them getting indignant, even when a good word would be helpful.

I sat back down next to my dad and whispered, "Dad, we know she shouldn't hit her kid that hard, but let's keep our comments to ourselves. We don't need anymore problems."

He scooted back on his mattress and lamented, "Yeah ... Okay, Son."

Not even 10 seconds later, some loud screaming and arguing came from behind us in the adjacent room. A highpitched female voice said something to the effect of, "You ain't gonna tell me what to mutha' fuckin' do! You ain't my daddy!"

A booming male voice yelled, "Fuck you bitch! I'll knock your ass out!"

She countered with, "I ain't scared of your punk ass! Fuck you! Come on mutha' fuck ..."

This couple's gonna come to blows in a minute.

My dad said, "What the hell is all that about?"

"I don't know, but it doesn't sound good."

A few seconds later, the female, whom I now realized was the medical clerk who works on the 10th floor, walked through the doorway with her one-year-old son in her arms shouting, "You ain't gonna fuck with me! You bitch ass nigger! You fuckin' with the wrong one!"

Later I found out the man she was arguing with was just somebody who had set up near them, and they were arguing about the space between them when the man began to threaten her.

I knew we were on the verge of everyone cracking. The heat was starting to affect everyone, and tempers were continuing to flare. I decided to grab my book, the latest *Harry Potter*, to try to pass the time by reading. It was getting late, and I wasn't too confident we would be leaving that day. They were still evacuating the inmates to the Broad Street Bridge and then to buses below the bridges. I grabbed a nearby chair and moved it close to the shattered window and began to read. I only had about a 100 pages left, and I figured I would read until it got close to dusk. My dad laid back and turned his face toward the wall. I put the book down for a minute, grabbed my pillows, and fanned him until he fell asleep.

Once he was snoring again, I sat back down and read. I tried to engross myself in the book so I could escape the horrendous predicament I was in. I kind of lost track of time and eventually went to sleep too.

I woke up later with the book lying in my lap. I looked at my dad and all I could see was the right side of his face and body. It didn't look like he was breathing. I got that nervous feeling in my chest again and watched his face for what seemed like an eternity.

Again, just when panic set in, he took a deep snoring breath through his nose and momentarily opened his eyes real wide, with his cheek quivering. He reached up and scratched his head and saw me looking at him. "What's wrong? Why are you looking at me?"

Relieved and startled at the same time, I said, "Oh, um ... I thought for a second that you had stopped breathing."

Half awake he said, "What? Why did you think that?"

"I've noticed over the past couple of days, when you're sleeping, sometimes you go a long time without breathing, and I thought that you had stopped breathing. Just as I was going to check your pulse or something, you took a deep snore through your nose and woke up."

He looked at me for a second or two and said, "I didn't know I did that."

"How could you? You're sleeping."

Chuckling, he said, "I guess you're right, Son. I'm all right though." With that, I got up and grabbed my water bottle and took a swig.

Evening was upon us, and there was no indication we would be leaving. It looked like another sweltering night in this cesspool. With the prospect of another night in there, I encouraged my dad to drink as much water as he could. I also suggested we prepare the MRE we had. "Hey Dad, are you hungry? We can fix this lasagna pack thing here, whatever it is."

"Yeah, I guess I could try it."

When I opened it up, I saw the directions on how to heat the lasagna. I have to say this was pretty neat. First, I took out the lasagna plate and then took the box and placed it on a flat surface (the floor).

Then there were those black packets that looked like gun powder or black sand I placed under the lasagna plate, which, when a small amount of water is put in the packets, activates the black powder instantly, producing steam and making the water boil. Next, we folded the outer edges of the box over the lasagna plate and let it "cook" for 12 to 14 minutes.

How would military people have 14 minutes to wait for the food to heat if they were engaged in some sort of battle — or was this a civilian type of MRE just for a situation like ours?

My dad and I watched the steam coming from the side and top of this box. After a couple of minutes, we had a few people standing by us watching this meal percolate.

"How long it takes to cook?" came from my left.

"About 12 to 14 minutes according to the directions," I answered.

Someone else was asking me about the meal preparation. "Is that steam? Where's that coming from?"

I grabbed the top portion of the box and showed them the directions. "Just follow the directions right here. It's real easy."

Looking at the box for a second with a tinge of confusion on his face he said, "Oh, thanks man. Let me go and try that."

By this time, our meal was ready. Because of the heat, I wasn't really hungry, but I knew I had better eat something. "Ready to eat, Pops?"

"Yeah, do we have to use our hands or what?"

"No, there's a fork here with the MRE for you to use. Here you go. Enjoy!"

The food was still pretty hot and his first bite nearly fell out of his mouth. A few seconds later I said, "I bet you never thought you'd be eating military lasagna sitting on the floor of a jail, in your underwear, huh, Dad?"

With his mouth half full, he said, "Nope. Can't say that I did."

"Is it good?"

"Not bad, Son; here, try some." He handed me his fork and I took a bite. Surprisingly, it really wasn't too bad. I took another bite or two, and gave the fork back to my dad. "Finish it off, Dad; I'll eat a little later."

"You sure?"

"Go ahead."

"You don't have any more M&Ms, do you?"

"No, I gave them to you earlier, but I'll see if I can trade something with somebody for some more M&Ms."

"Thanks."

"Hey, Dad, I'll be back in a minute. I'm going to go see if I can find anything out about when we'll be leaving here."

He casually replied, "See you later."

When I got to the roof, the sun was beginning to creep down toward the horizon. It was another beautiful day (except for the heat) without a cloud in the sky. The orange-blue sunset was becoming all too familiar. There were plenty of people on the roof, many of them getting prepared to sleep outside for the night. There were mattresses set up all over, and it would definitely be cooler at night up there than inside. I also think the smell of the building inside had gotten unbearable to most folks. If I had been by myself, I would have been sleeping outside too.

After wandering around the roof for a while, I noticed the helicopter activity had slowed down, and I was hearing fewer boats moving around on the water. I didn't know if that meant there were fewer people to evacuate or because night was approaching, and with no lights in the city, they were going to shut it down for the night. I took one last look at the Broad Street Bridge, and there were still plenty of stranded civilians and a few inmates left. We might not be leaving that day, but we had to be getting close. Four days was enough.

I looked over toward the Templeman Buildings and didn't see any inmates waving white sheets or towels for help or sitting on the rooftops anymore. I asked one of the deputies if he heard any news.

"Man, I don't know! Anywhere but here is fine with me."

I was about to go back downstairs when I almost ran into Robert at the entrance to the roof. I said, "Just who I was looking for. Robert, are we leaving tomorrow?"

"Gavin, I'm fairly confident we will, but you know, who knows?" He shrugged his shoulders. "Be prepared to leave though. Remember, you can only bring one bag, if they let you take anything at all, that is."

"Yeah, I remember. See you later."

Back on the second floor, the scene was familiar. People of all walks of life lumped together, worn out, overheated, sitting or lying down, sleeping or dazed, listening to the few remaining radios with working batteries. It was getting dark inside and when I got over to my dad, I noticed someone had lit the candle. My dad was lying down with his hands behind his head just looking up at the ceiling.

"Hey, Dad, it looks like tomorrow."

Not even looking at me and with a sarcastic tone he said, "I'll believe it when I see it."

"Me too, but I heard that they're going to move the elderly and sick people first."

Defiantly, he replied, "Well, I'm not sick, Son, so that doesn't do us any good."

Laughing to myself I said, "Yeah, but you're elderly I know everyone thinks you're 50, but you technically fall under the elderly category."

"Yeah, but ..." He must have thought about it for a second and said, "Hey, whatever gets us outta here will work for me."

Smiling at him, I said, "Now you're thinking. Just go along with me, and we'll be outta here soon.""

At that moment, someone was letting the bathroom door slam again: "BAM!"

"Damn door. I wish I had a dollar for every time that damn door slammed closed."

"I hear ya, Dad. I just wish when the door slammed the smell would get slammed out of the building."

"No kidding!" And we both laughed a little.

By this point, there wasn't much I could do on the 10th floor, but I knew I had to go up there for a little while, just in case something happened. I told my dad I would be back in a little while.

I could see the disappointed look on his face when I told him I'd be leaving.

"I guess I'll be here tonight — again."

I shook my head yes and said, "See you in a little bit," and began my way upstairs. I took one last look at him before I turned around. He was lying down, facing the wall again.

I got to the stairs and realized I didn't have my flashlight. I went to go back and took a few steps. Ah, screw it. I decided to walk the stairs in the dark. I figured by this point, all the inmates were evacuated, and there were no more wolf-dogs in the building. It took me several minutes to walk the stairs, and I imagined what it must be like to be blind.

Once I got to the 10th floor, covered in sweat, I couldn't believe how quiet and dark it was. No one was up there and everyone, including the inmates, was either on the roof, on the second floor, or evacuated. Since I was already on 10, I tried to make a phone call. After a couple of attempts with no success, I text-messaged Lora saying, "I LUV U. STILL HERE. HOPE 2 SEE U SOON. GAV." I got the confirmation it went through and took one last look outside, figuring it might be the last time I would do so. I didn't think I would be back. With all the rumored devastation to most of the building and the city, my time there was hopefully almost over. After contemplating for a few minutes, I made my way back downstairs, making a pit stop on the roof to see what was going on and to get one last bit of fresh air before going to my spot for the night.

The roof was bursting with people and activity. The word was spreading we'd be leaving in the morning, around 8 a.m. All the inmates from the entire system were evacuated with our building, HOD, being the last (of course). Although we were going to be the last ones evacuated, I could hear, for the first time, some optimism in everyone's voices. "Are they really getting here?"

"Man, I thought they forgot about us!"

"I can't wait to get out of here!"

It seemed everyone on the roof had an opinion about when, where, and how we would be moved the next day.

I thought I would walk over to the side of the roof to see if the woman with the sign was still stranded. It was dark outside, except for the moon and billions of stars above, and a few flashlights shining about. I looked where I first saw her, but it was too dark to see anything. After a minute or two of straining my eyes to see anything, I gave up and went back downstairs. Maybe she'd gotten out safely.

Everyone on the second floor looked exhausted or was sleeping. The mood down there was not as animated as on the roof. When I got near my dad, he was talking to Dr. Marcus and Nurse Urban.

"What's up guys?" I asked.

My dad said, "Where you been, Son?"

"I was on 10 for a few minutes and then on the roof for a little while — I have good news! We're supposed to be leaving in the morning around 8 a.m."

"Yeah, I heard that one before."

Dr. Marcus said, "Oh really? That's great!"

Urban said, "I really believe we will leave tomorrow ... I just don't know if it will be as early as they say."

For the next hour or so, we all sat around talking, sweating, sipping on water, still in disbelief we were in this horrible situation. Our little candle was lit, giving off the comforting light. As the conversations slowed down, I found myself lying back, peacefully watching the candle flicker.

Unfortunately, our respite was short-lived. Nearby someone had a radio on, and the news was still the same. The looting and raging fires seemed to dominate the airwaves, along with the reports of dead bodies and the water still rising in the city.

After some thought, I just prayed in the direction of the candle for a variety of things. First and foremost, for my dad's safety and health. As I prayed, the candle seemed to get brighter, and I got chills again — yes, real chills — down my entire body. In the midst of all this chaos and suffering, I really began to feel like maybe we were going to be all right.

I grabbed my pillow to fan my dad so he could go to sleep. The sooner he fell asleep, the sooner tomorrow would come, and hopefully we would be out of there. When he gave out a little snore every 10 seconds or so, I knew he was okay. It took me a while to fall asleep; well, I really never was completely at rest because I kept catching myself checking on him to make sure he was still breathing.

The last time I looked at my phone, it was around midnight. I turned it off to save the battery, because there was no way to charge it. I was only awake from pure adrenaline. My body was exhausted, but my mind was still racing. Would we get out of here soon? Where would we live? Where would I work? I don't have a car. My dad's car is gone. What will I do with my dad?

Where's my mom? Is my little brother alive?

On and on my mind kept racing with questions. I worried myself to sleep.

Chapter 15

Evacuation

POP-POP-POP, POW, POW, POW!!

More gunfire woke me up. A hint of daylight shone through the window, but no one else was awake. I looked over at my father and right on cue he gave a little snore. I was completely soaked in sweat. Going on my fifth day without a shower (if you don't count that ice cold, one minute shower I took late Sunday night), my body odor was really starting to be noticeable. I started having daydreams of taking a two-hour bubble bath with my honey massaging my back and feeding me chocolate-covered strawberries or something.

Back to my reality. I grabbed my towel, which by then was pretty smelly too, and a little water and wiped myself down. I was starving and felt pretty weak, and I took a couple bites of a granola bar.

I noticed how hauntingly quiet it was inside and out. For the past couple days, the helicopters and flat boats had filled the air with loud whirring sounds, making it seem like a war zone. Stretching back out and imagining a better place to be, I must have fallen asleep again.

The next thing I knew, my dad was nudging me and whispering, "Gavin... Son... I gotta go to the bathroom." Same story, different day.

Once we finished, I changed into the last clean shirt I had and put on some shorts. It was sizzling hot already, but I didn't want to walk around in my underwear. I gave my dad one of my not-too-dirty T-shirts so he could wipe the sweat off himself.

"Well, Son, I hope this is the day!"

Feeling optimistic, I exclaimed, "Me too, Dad! Hopefully, this morning sometime. Just be ready."

I got up and made my way to the roof. It was another beautiful clear day, and only a few people milled around. Some were talking while others were sitting under the ledge out of the sun. I saw Nurse Robert standing by the entrance to the parking garage looking out over the ledge.

Making my way over to him, I overheard someone say, "They were supposed to be here by 8 a.m. Where are they?"

I asked someone standing nearby what the time was and they said it was 8:20.

Damn! I don't see any signs of boats.

I made my way over to Robert and asked, "What's up?"

With a somewhat guilty look on his face he said, "I don't know.

They were supposed to be here by 8 o'clock, and I don't see them anywhere."

"Who's they?"

"The D. O. C., I was told. Fuckin' I don't know. All I can tell you is that they know we're here, and somebody's gonna come and get us. Just be ready!" I could see he had probably been asked the same questions a thousand times, and I had asked a bunch.

Dejected, I took my time walking back downstairs. I decided not to say anything to my dad or for that matter to anyone else. It was only about 8:45. I saw a few nurses standing in the main hallway and stopped by them to chat for a little while. Nurse Favis and Nurse Tech Michelle were leaning against the wall talking.

"Can y'all believe this? It's Friday and we're still here," I said.

"We gotta get outta here soon. This is unbearable," Favis said.

"How's your dad? Is he all right?" Michelle asked.

"Okay, as far as I can tell. Thanks for asking. By the way, how is your finger? Does it still hurt?" "It's real stiff and a pretty sore, but not too bad."

"Keep takin' those antibiotics and you should be all right. If I hear anything about leavin', I'll let y'all know," I said as I walked away.

It was after 9 a.m., and I still didn't hear sounds of boats. I did hear an occasional helicopter flying around the area though. I found my dad lying down, fanning himself with my pillow.

"What's up, Dad?"

"My blood pressure, I'm sure. I have one pill left ... are we going home soon or what?"

After all of this time I thought I had made it clear that going home was not an option. Did he really think we were going home? I waited a few seconds before I said anything. Going on a hunch and a prayer I said, "We're being moved out of here first to dry land and then we'll have to see about home. I know my house is flooded, and we can't go there. I don't know about your house yet. Let's just concentrate on getting outta here first."

He didn't say anything and neither did I. I didn't want to upset him. I felt like a broken record and wasn't quite sure where my dad's physical and mental state was.

The time was passing painfully slowly now and with the heat everyone was in slow motion. Nine a.m. became 10 and 10 became 11. I was really hungry, but I forced myself not to eat. I decided to take a walk toward the main hallway near the exit to the inmate's recreational area. I was walking slowly with my head down when all of the sudden Robert came through the second-floor stairwell door yelling, "Sick and elderly people, let's go! There are some boats ready to go! Sick and elderly people, let's …"

As I turned around, Robert walked fast toward me and said, "Get your bag and your dad and get to the roof. Now! Hurry!"

Caught by surprise, I ran back over to my dad and said, "Put your shoes, socks, and pants on — we're outta here!" He was lying down and half out of it. "Come on, Dad, we're leaving!"

"Are we going home?"

"Dad, get up and get dressed. We have to go to the roof now!"

Helping him get his stuff together, I put on my socks and tennis shoes and zipped up both bags. Since I had stuffed them full, they were heavy. I helped him stand up and get his balance. For the first time in a while we both smiled at each other, knowing that we were getting out of there. "Come on, Dad, I'll carry both bags! Your left shoe is untied. Tie it real quick!"

The stairwell was still quite dark. I had a bag on each shoulder and told him to hold the handrail and the bag on my right shoulder. "Follow me slowly up the stairs. We only have to go one and a half flights of stairs, and then we'll go through a door that will lead to the roof!"

Confused, he said, "Why are we going to the roof?"

"Just follow me. You'll see!"

Once we were on the roof, there were about 10 or 12 people with us who fell under the sick and elderly category. Nurse Donna was with her husband (who recently had to retire due to poor health); Deputy Harriet and her uncle, who had a history of strokes and needed help walking; Ms. Cece, a rank official, had her mother who needed to be moved, as she needed dialysis.

The individual who needed medical attention most urgently was Deputy Lee. He was a tall black man in his mid- to late-30s who had diabetes and had injured his big toe during the aftermath. He had gone a few days without his insulin, and his feet were starting to swell, causing him to walk with an obvious limp. I asked, "What happened?"

He looked at me grimacing and said, "Man, I don't even remember. All I know is that the pain in my foot is killing me!"

As we all stood by the doorway that led us one step closer to freedom, I saw Captain Brumfield and asked him how bad the building was. "Well G, I don't see us back here for a long time — at least a year. Half of those buildings have holes in the walls where the inmates tried to escape. All the Templeman buildings are probably destroyed. CCC is real fucked up too. Don't worry about comin' back here any time soon. It's been nice workin' with ya, G — good luck!"

Shaking his hand I said, "All right, Cap, take it easy. Good luck!" I stood there for a minute, realizing that my time there was finally ending, but it was the first time I realized for exactly how long. My feelings were foggy. Relief. Sadness. Confusion. They called to us to walk through the doorway.

We made our way to the parking garage that connected to the roof and down the ramp to the bottom level. The water was a good way up the bottom level ramp, at least seven to eight feet or so. There were two flat boats and another boat. Once we got to the bottom level, we filed into each boat. There were three or four deputies helping those who needed it. Each boat was surrounded by all kinds of debris — sticks, trash, paper, a couple tires — just about anything I could think of. Everyone was trying to get on the boats too fast, frustrating the individuals navigating the boats.

"We're going to have to make a couple of trips, so everyone just be patient."

I had my dad sit down on the curb that ran up the driveway. "Let's just wait for the second trip. The bridge isn't that far away, and there's no use in hurrying up now. We'll just be on that bridge in the heat anyway."

"That's fine, Son. At least we're sort of moving."

People stepped up on a little piece of concrete sticking up out of the water to get into the boats. The only problem was one of the boats was much higher than the other. I noticed a strong gasoline smell.

One of the deputies said, "All those motorcycles and cars up there were being siphoned off for gas — that's what they've been running the boats off of." Looking up, I saw a row of police motorcycles and cars. Thank God those vehicles were there because they were the only source of gasoline available.

After about 15 minutes, one of the boats came back. It was a different-looking boat. It pulled up as close as it could, and a man yelled to us, "Let's go! You two!"

I grabbed both bags and my dad got up, losing his balance a little. We got as close as we could to the boat without stepping into the water.

Deputy Stan, a tall, strapping young African-American, was standing in the water with boots on. He and I worked on the 10th floor from time to time, and he kept order up there better than any other deputy. Stan turned to my dad and said, "Come on, Pops, I got ya." With that, he stepped toward my dad and picked him up like he was a bag of groceries and put him in the boat. It was funny to watch because my dad is a pretty tall man. I tossed each bag on the boat, stepped on the section of cement and got in. My feet got wet, and I had thoughts of contamination covering them. As I positioned myself in the front of the boat, we backed up out of the garage and went down the street, navigating carefully around the cars and trash in the water. The Broad Street Bridge was about 200 yards away, and as we approached the bridge we pulled up right next to the circular on-ramp. I threw the bags over the guardrail, stepped up on and then over the rail and onto the concrete on-ramp.

My dad stepped across the boat on the edge, and I grabbed him under his arm while the man in the boat pushed him up and I pulled him over the guardrail. We slowly walked up the ramp on to the upslope of the bridge. "Well, we're out of there, thank God!"

I could see my dad was a little disoriented and really didn't know what to say.

We walked over to where the others were and sat down. It was hot as hell, and the sun felt like it was beating down directly on us. The deputy with the bad toe had his shoe off looking at his foot. I walked over to him and right away noticed his big toe was split on the outside below the nail, but there was no blood. It was also quite swollen and greenish in color. He looked at me and said, "Whatcha' think, Doc? This sonofabitch is hurtin' real bad." When

I looked at it, I instantly knew that it didn't look good. It appeared to have gangrene and needed immediate medical attention. He might well lose that toe.

"Man, you need to get medical assistance ASAP. Try to stay off of that foot as much as possible."

He looked away and then back at me and said, "Am I gonna lose my toe or what?"

Trying to stay positive, I said, "I don't know. Do you know where we are going from here? If you can get medical attention soon, I think it will be all right."

"Hey, I stepped in a lot of that dirty water ... you think it'll be okay?" I figured the toxic water probably contributed to his condition.

"I don't know man. Let me get a bottle of water and we'll clean it off."

I went over to one of my bags and got a fresh, unopened bottle of water and one of my T-shirts. I poured the water over his toe and tried to clean it as best as I could while he clenched his teeth in pain.

I finished cleaning his toe and gave him my T-shirt to wrap around his foot. Meanwhile, my dad was starting to wander up the bridge, and there were a lot of rough-looking characters walking around near him. I didn't want him to get into any trouble, so I yelled, "Hey Dad, come here!" He turned around, and I waved him toward me.

A military helicopter flew over us and circled around, landing in the middle of the bridge. We were sitting about 100 yards or so from where the helicopter landed, and the wind generated from the propellers was furious.

Everyone around us started talking. *Are we supposed to be getting on the helicopter or what?* In the opposite direction, we were surrounded by water and in the distance down Broad Street, some boats headed our way. No one told us anything when we were evacuating the House of Detention building, and we had no idea what to do or where we were going. It was beyond frustrating.

I told my dad to sit down next to Deputy Lee. "I'm gonna go up to the top of the bridge to see if I can find out where the heck we're going." I got up and walked quickly to the top of the bridge. There were maybe about 200 people, predominantly black, elderly, and most looked somewhat ill. The dismay and desperation on everyone's faces will always be burned in my memory.

At the top of the bridge was a rope tied from one side of the bridge to the other. There were about three or four black men ranging from about 16 years of age to about 40. They were directing people toward the helicopter that had just landed on the bridge and helping those people get into the chopper. I eventually got one of them to come over to me so I could ask them where the helicopters were going, if we were to get on them, whether we should get on the boats, things like that.

The helicopter was just taking off stirring up a tremendous amount of wind, dust and trash. I yelled, "Do you know where we're supposed to go?!"

Squinting his eyes from the wind, he yelled back, "To the airport; sick first, then the elderly!" He then pointed to an area across from me to my left saying, "There is the line! You got any sick or old people with you?"

I turned around and pointed to our group at the bottom of the bridge and said, "Yes! Some sick; one real bad. And some elderly!"

The man pointed again to the line and said, "Get in line!"

As I walked back down the bridge, I saw an abandoned car casting some shade to its side. I decided to go get my dad and let him lie down on my bag in the shade so he wouldn't overheat.

When I got down to everybody, I said, "The helicopters are going to the airport, bringing sick and elderly first. We have to get in line and as the helicopters land, we'll be directed to get on them."

Donna said, "What about the boats? Where are they going?"

Realizing I didn't think to ask about the boats, I said, "It was so loud I didn't even ask. I figured the airport wouldn't be that bad, and they were getting the sick and elderly off the bridge first."

Deputy Lee started to stand up and lost his balance a little, so I helped him up. As he gained his balance, with great determination he said, "I'm going to get in that line. I gotta get my toe looked at as soon as possible."

As the group started to talk about what to do, I walked my dad over to the abandoned car and said, "Sit here, out of the sun until we can get on one of those helicopters."

"Where are they going to bring us? Home?"

Agitated and saddened by my dad's denial of the situation, I said, "Dad, we don't have a home to go home to. The helicopters are bringing people to the airport. Sick and elderly people first."

He nervously asked, "You're gonna be with me, right?"

"Of course, Dad. We're in this together until it's over." I had to force back tears.

I went back up toward the top of the bridge to watch for another helicopter. The men directing the people on the bridge formed another line for "immediate needs" individuals and as I heard them talking, I ran back down to gather everybody up. "Hey y'all, they're making another line for immediate needs individuals to fly out to the airport. Let's get in line!"

Everybody stood up, some faster than others, and began to walk up the bridge. Deputy Harriet's uncle was having a hard time, so I grabbed his bag for him. I was now walking up the bridge with three bags, one on each shoulder and one in my hands, like an overloaded hotel bellman or something.

Once we got to the top of the bridge, there wasn't much organization, and I could see people were going to be aggressive in their attempts to get on the helicopters. The next one was in the process of landing as we sat down in line. One of the "guys in charge" was a young, African-American kid about 16 or 17 years old with no shirt on and his shorts hanging halfway off his butt. "All right, ya'll, listen up! I'll wave y'all forward when the chopper lands ... only two or three at a time. Keep ya heads down, ya heard me?"

This is unbelievable. We have a half-dressed teenager directing a military evacuation after a major disaster. No one would believe me if I told them this!

I helped Deputy Lee with his stuff to the front of the line yelling, "I am a nurse, and this man needs to get out of here! On this chopper! He needs immediate medical attention or he will lose his toe!"

"All right. All right. When they give me the signal, he can go!"

A deputy and I looked at each other and laughed for a second. I'm sure he was thinking the same thing I was thinking, Look at this kid running the show! Unbelievable!

After a minute or so, the military person in the helicopter made a hand gesture and our "leader" motioned for Deputy Lee to come forward. I grabbed his bag and helped him to the chopper, fighting the hurricane-force wind from the blades. Once he was safely in, I went back by my dad, barely keeping my balance and standing over him, covering his face to protect him from all the trash and dust flying all over the place. A couple people from our group got on the helicopter along with a few other people who needed immediate attention. I yelled to my dad, "We'll wait for the next one, okay?"

He nodded in agreement, and I kept protecting his face until the helicopter flew off.

About five minutes later, another chopper landed on the bridge, and this time it was rushed by a crowd of people. It was becoming a dog-eat-dog situation. I told my dad we would wait for a couple more helicopters, since they seemed to be coming with regularity. "There's no use in fighting the crowd right now. We're in line to get out of here before a lot of these people who have been on this bridge longer than us."

At this point I could see he was worn out. We both were. I approached Deputy Harriet and her uncle and suggested we stick together and I would help her with her uncle. "That's fine, Gavin. We'll go when y'all go."

There were about eight of us left, and I stood up and said, "We'll catch one of the next couple of helicopters." Everyone nodded in agreement. I went to one of the guys directing traffic and said, "Our group right here will try and all get on together. We have a few people who need medical attention, but nothing that is an emergency."

"All right, bra'. We'll try for the next one," he said.

We nodded thank you.

About 10 minutes later, another chopper landed and we got up together and waited for the signal. I grabbed our bags and Deputy Harriet's uncle's bag. I put my hand on top of my dad's head and told him, "Keep your head down as we approach the helicopter!"

We ambled purposefully as the wind from the blades nearly knocked us down. I threw the bags in the helicopter toward an empty seat in the back, then helped my dad step up on to the floor-board to the last empty seat. Then I helped Harriet's uncle on to the floor of the helicopter, and I sat on the floor right in front of my dad. All the while, the noise from the chopper blades was deafening.

There was a seatbelt that came down over both of my dad's shoulders and hooked into a center buckle that came from under the seat. There was also a circular buckle that locked from both sides. I could see my dad was struggling with figuring out how it worked. I halfway turned around and hooked it together for him.

He smiled and I yelled, "We're finally out of this nightmare!"

The entire floor of the helicopter was filled with maybe 15 to 20 people, most of whom were sitting on the floor. Everyone had a nervous look on his or her faces.

There were two military guys in the front and another guy in the back with us. They all had helmets and sunglasses on and looked quite intimidating, but were very friendly. Those guys were the best.

The one in the back with us made a hand gesture to the pilot and then to the guys on the ground as they backed up from the helicopter. About 10 seconds later, we started to lift off the ground, and I got that "tickling butterflies" sensation in my stomach that I'd only had on a roller coaster before. My dad was smiling, so I guess he was feeling the same sensation I was. We went straight up, then dipped down and started to fly north, toward Lake Pontchartrain. I had never been on a helicopter, and this ride was truly amazing. I'm not quite sure what type of helicopter it was, but it was black, fast, and modern-looking. It may have been a Blackhawk or something close to it.

Flying toward the lake, I looked out to my right, and I could see that the entire area right off of the I-10 Interstate (the highway included) was completely under water. We veered to the left, and I could see where the levee had broken at the Seventeenth Street Canal. What a sight. A fateful, dreadful sight.

The next second I looked to my left and there was no floodwater anywhere. It was very strange to see all that water to the east side of the canal, but no water to the west. It appeared the Metairie side of the canal didn't break. All I saw was house after house with roof damage, trees down everywhere, signs scattered all over the streets, cars strewn everywhere, but no signs of people at all. Strange, strange and ghostly, actually.

It dawned on me we were flying in the direction of my home in Kenner, so I waited a few seconds, and I tried to look toward where I lived. As far as I could tell the flooding was down or gone. I couldn't see my condominium, but the destruction in the area was quite evident. Soon we turned and started our descent to the airport.

I could see people unloading from numerous helicopters, all in a line by a long runway strip. As we landed, I saw the vehicles airlines use to move luggage on to planes. We landed just about how we took off and rolled up in a perfect line behind a number of other helicopters. It was a 10-minute flight I will never forget, and I'm sure my dad won't either.

As I went to step off of the helicopter, I nearly fell down because I had no feeling in my right foot. I guess someone had been sitting on it. After helping Deputy Harriet's uncle and a few others down, I jumped back up into the chopper and helped my dad get unhooked and off the helicopter. Waiting for us was one of the luggage vehicles. We were directed to sit on the side of one of them. I threw our bags in the middle, helped my dad up on to the side, and hopped in.

A wave of emotions hit me when we started to move, and tears welled up in my eyes. The reality we were finally out of that nightmare situation and on dry land coupled with the fact my dad was still alive hit me hard. Real hard.

What's next?

When we went toward the main area of the airport, I could see what looked like hundreds of people standing, sitting, or walking around. The odd thing was it looked like most people could hardly move. A few minutes or so later we pulled up to an unloading area near a gate, and all I saw was a turbulent sea of people – all kinds of harried people. On one side, I saw an area that looked like a M.A.S.H. medical unit.

We were told to go through an open gate, and as we started to walk, an elderly man with a walker shuffling along started to fall.

I gave one of the bags to my dad and helped this old man slowly walk through the gate and over to the makeshift medical area.

My dad walked straight ahead through the gate and sat down on the curb under the down-ramp of the second level of the airport. This appeared to be an area where most of the people were going. A military medical person met me at the entrance to the medical unit.

"What is his medical problem?"

"I don't know sir; I was just helping him walk from the dropoff area." The elderly man stood silent with his head bowed.

"I'll take it from here. Thanks."

I walked over and sat down by my dad. Exhausted and relieved. "Well, Buddy, at least we're on dry land and out of the city!"

My dad looked at me and asked, "Now what?"

I just looked around at the crowd of people wandering around. Just about everyone looked disoriented or confused. I asked my dad to sit down and said I would walk around to see if anyone knew what was going on. As I stood up, I saw a gigantic African-American man struggling to walk through the gate leading to where we were. The man was in obvious pain.

There were people walking right by him, not offering any help. I stood there for a few seconds and watched him try to walk. He wore what looked like work boots, shorts, and a torn T-shirt. He was well over 300 pounds and well over 6 feet tall.

Once I realized no one was with him or was going to help him, I went over and offered, "Hey Buddy, you need some help?" He looked surprised someone was willing to help him.

"Well, Yes. Thanks. Thank you, Son." I could see his legs were swollen and his feet were in immense pain by the way he was walking. I asked him, "What's wrong with your feet?" With what looked like all the energy he had left, he said, "I have diabetes, and my feet have sores on them. I haven't had my medicine in a few days." I figured he probably had foot ulcers.

Trying to reassure him, I said, "Well, sir, they have some sort of medical area set up over there. If you want, I can help you over there to see if they can help you."

"Man, I would appreciate that."

I got on the left side of this gargantuan man and put my right arm around his waist and told him to lean on my right shoulder and try to walk. It took us an agonizingly long time to walk about 50 yards to the medical area. When we finally reached it, I shouted, "This man is a diabetic and needs immediate medical attention!"

One of the nurses turned around and ran toward an area where they had transport vehicles and the other nurse or doctor said, "We got him."

The man turned to me and shook my hand saying, "Thanks man. Thank you." His eyes reddened with gratitude.

Smiling, I said, "You're welcome. Good luck, man."

I looked to my left and saw the deputy with the bad toe being helped through a doorway on the side of the main building. I hoped he'd be all right.

I walked toward the main doorway to the bottom level of the airport. There were people lying on the ground, sitting against the wall, walking around, talking, arguing, eating, sleeping — anything imaginable. I went further and all I saw were more people and more calamity. I walked up to someone who looked like they might work there and said, "Can you tell me what to do or where to go?" The guy looked agitated and pointed up toward the escalators and stairs that were filled with people. I stood there for a second, looking at everyone fighting their way to get up the stairs and decided to wait a little while and go up there later.

I went back over by my dad and saw him buying some cigarettes from a drunk-looking guy. I was going to say something, but decided not to. I could see the stress on my dad's face, so I figured if he thought he needed a cigarette, he should have one. I sat back down next to him, and we had our group together from the HOD.

There was an area right next to the medical area where some people were putting bottles and bottles of water into a huge "pool looking" structure filled with ice behind a loose chain-link fence. I immediately got up, pointed and told everyone, "Hey, look, they're giving out water over there. Let's get some!" A few of us walked over there and grabbed some bottles of water. Word spread fast and mobs of people started attacking the bottled water pool. We got ours and got out of the way. Those in charge realized they had to create some order, so they closed the chain-link gate and started handing water over the fence to people who needed or asked for it. Of course, there were people taking advantage and getting more than they needed.

About 15 minutes later, a forklift came from out of nowhere with a crate full of MREs. A couple of military individuals stood by us as the crate was lowered to the ground and MREs were handed out. I got in line and got one each for my dad and me. This would be our first full meal in a few days. I went back over to the curb and ripped open the MRE to see what I could eat. I gobbled up a bag of trail mix real quick. My main meal was a vegetarian one and my dad's was beef with mushrooms.

I was super hungry, and the MRE tasted like filet mignon to me! As we ate, the guy my dad bought the cigarettes from was lying face down on the concrete passed out. All of a sudden, he started coughing and jerking around a little. He then started dry heaving and about 30 seconds later started vomiting. He was obviously drunk or on some kind of illicit drugs. He woke up and stood up while everybody in the immediate area jumped up and got out of his way. He looked around for a few seconds and said, in an impaired manner, "I'm all right, yeah, yeah, I'm good!" while wiping the puke from his face. Everyone watching started to giggle a bit as the man staggered around and wandered off.

Due to the smelly mess he made near us, we decided to slide down the curb a little way. I went over to where they were handing out water and poured a few bottles over the vomit to help wash it away. Once we got resettled, I finished eating, although it wasn't as appealing as it was before. I told our group I was going to go up to the upper level to see what our next move would be. I walked back over to the escalator and stairs area and maneuvered my way up. The upper level of the Louis Armstrong International Airport is where you go to check in for a flight, and it has all sorts of restaurants, shops, a video arcade, etc.; of course, all closed up. As I stepped off the last step to the second floor, I was stunned at what I saw – thousands and thousands of people packed together wandering about. I could barely walk forward from the top step and didn't know which way to go. I stepped to my right to get out of the way, but that was virtually impossible.

Frantically, people walked and ran into each other, crying and yelling in outright bedlam. I saw what looked like an airport employee and fought through the crowd toward him, getting bumped and knocked around in the process. Once I got to him, I yelled, "Do you know what we're supposed to do? I just got here a short time ago!"

It took this guy a second to catch his breath and then he said, as he pointed behind me, "You have to get in line over there to get registered to get on a plane to somewhere, either San Antonio, Austin, Dallas, somewhere like that!"

I turned around and my heart sank in my chest. There was a line that extended for as far as I could see filled with people crying, screaming, talking loudly, and yelling.

I turned back to the man and asked, "Is that the only way outta here?!"

Apologetically, he answered, "Yes! But from that line you have to get into that line to get on a plane, and you don't have a choice as to where you go. I've heard people will be on military bases for a month or so!"

Just as I turned back to ask the man something else, an older man fell over, hit the ground, and appeared to have a seizure. The man I was talking to instantly grabbed a walkietalkie and said, "I need medical backup by the main escalator! Man down! I repeat – I need backup!"

At this point I didn't know what to do. By law, I am a nurse and if I initiate treatment on this guy I can become liable if something goes wrong, but I couldn't let this guy lie there and not do anything. His wife, I guess, started crying hysterically, so I told her to help me turn him on his side and she needed to hold him there until help came. I got down and turned the man on his side, making sure his head was parallel to the floor, and told the woman to hold him as steady as she could until help came. The lady frantically said, "Oh! Are you a doctor?"

"No ma'am. Just do it!" As I got up to walk away, she thanked me, and I didn't even look back. I walked toward the back of the first line, and it went on forever. I turned to look at the second line and saw it was worse. It was so loud and crowded, I decided to go toward the sliding glass doors that led to the outside of the second level.

Pacing outside, I tried to compose myself, as I could feel anxiety and panic building. I tried to breathe slow, deep breaths.

Looking left, I saw a convoy of military vehicles unloading people. To my right, I saw a row of yellow port-a-lets and a few armed military personnel guys directing traffic. Down toward the end, to the right, I saw a tall, broad-shouldered Caucasian army soldier with a gun, standing by himself. I decided to go over to him to see if he had any ideas as to what was going to happen.

I walked up to him and asked, "Have you ever seen anything like this before?"

He looked at me for a second, curled a smile, and said, "I was in Iraq for over a year, and I never saw anything close to this. This is unbelievable! This is something like out of a movie. It's crazy!"

I waited a second or two before I asked, "What should I do? I have my 83-year-old dad with me, and he's out of his medicine.

They're saying inside we have to get on a plane and fly to Texas, but they don't know where."

He was half-joking and half-serious, I guess, when he replied, "Man, if I were you I would go try and steal a car or something and drive the hell out of here!" He paused for a couple of seconds and then said, "The only problem is they might stop you a few miles down the road at the checkpoint to see if the car is yours."

Smiling, he pointed and said, "Across the highway there (pointing to the south) I heard there are different police agencies; you might be able to find out something over there."

I stood there watching people unload from various military vehicles. I still didn't know what to do. I shook the guy's hand and thanked him. "Good luck," he said.

Another "good luck." Seemed to be a lot of those going around.

I shuffled back toward the sliding glass doors contemplating what to do. I did not want to get on some plane and go to a military base for who knew how long with my dad. *Would we be under Marshal Law? What exactly did that mean?* I couldn't see him making it through that scenario after all he'd been through so far. I looked up and saw, once again — total chaos. I decided I couldn't and wouldn't board a plane. I had to figure something out fast.

Getting knocked around like a pinball, I made my way back to the escalator and stairway where I had come from. I didn't walk 30 feet before another person keeled over, falling into the person next to him. I wanted to stop and help, but I had to keep going, to get my dad and me out of there. This happened two more times before I could get off the second level down to the ground level. It was more and more surreal. This can't be real! I must be dreaming!

Over near my dad and the others, I saw Deputy Rico and his family and a couple of nurses from the House of Detention building. They saw me and made their way over. "Hey Gavin. How long have you been here?"

Surprised to see them, I said, "Hey y'all! Not long, an hour or two. I'll tell you, though, this is as bad — if not worse — than where we were before! It's a freakin' mad house on the second level. They got people passing out, fighting to get in line! No one knows what the hell is goin' on!"

A few seconds later, some Louisiana State Police officers approached and asked Deputy Rico to show some identification because he had his firearm on his hip. Defensively, he said, "I'm an Orleans Parish deputy, and we just got here. I'm tryin' to find out what the hell is going on!"

One of the state officers then said, "You're gonna have to come with us and turn that gun in ... you can't walk around with it in this environment."

Turning back to me, he said, "Can you believe this shit? Do me a favor and tell my wife I'll be back in a minute!"

Shaking my head in disbelief, I said, "No problem. Don't worry, I'll tell 'em."

I saw his wife and kids about 50 yards away, but before I could get to them, Nurse Favis, her daughter, and Nurse Beatrice came up to me saying, "What's up G? We made it!"

I hastily said, "I don't know, this is pretty bad too. Have you been on the second level yet?"

They looked at each other and said, "Not yet ... why?" I proceeded to tell them about the frenzied scene up there and how if you get on a plane you would be flown to Texas somewhere with no definite plan.

"I ain't getting on no plane ... screw that!" Beatrice shouted.

Favis stood there blankly.

"Go take a look for yourself. If you decide to get on a plane, you better get in line now or there's no tellin' how long it will take to get outta here. Hey y'all, I'm going back over by my dad and the others so I can tell 'em what's going on." Pointing behind them toward the down ramp over the unruly crowd, I said, "I'll be over there until I figure out what to do. See y'all later."

As I walked back to my dad, all I saw were ailing people: people in wheelchairs, lying on tables with I.V. lines in their arms, and lying on the ground receiving medical care. I started to feel a slight bit better at the sight of this many people getting the medical care they needed.

I prayed silently my dad wouldn't end up in there.

Everyone in our area just looked dog-tired. Nurse Donna sipped on bottled water while wiping the sweat from her forehead as her husband leaned back on his bag, half asleep. My dad was standing up smoking a cigarette, still looking somewhat disoriented.

Deputy Harriet saw me and pulled me to the side saying, "Hey G, my uncle needs to go to the bathroom. Can you help me?"

Pointing up and behind us I said, "Yeah sure. The only bathrooms I saw were port-o-lets, outside on the second level."

She looked at me with a frustrated look. I added, "Let's go over to that medical area. I'm sure with your uncle's condition (partial paralysis from a stroke) they will help you. They must have a useable bathroom in there."

We got him up and helped him walk over to the medical unit, and they did take him in. Deputy Harriet went in with him and as she went to go in, she thanked me. I could see she was really worried about him, and I was happy to help her.

In the rush to evacuate her family, Deputy Harriet told me after everyone had evacuated, she realized no one had remembered to get her uncle, so she had to get him and bring him to the prison. She said, "Thank God I went and got him, because he lives in Gentilly (eastern New Orleans, near the lake). He probably would have drowned!"

Once she was inside with him, I walked back over to our spot and sat down for a minute to take a break. I needed to think about what to do. My house was only a couple miles from the airport and although I was sure it was flooded, maybe the upstairs portion was all right, just maybe. Could we stay up there? My main concern was the fact there was no electricity there and it would be very hot. It was starting to seem more appealing to fly out of there.

I eventually stood to get everyone's attention, "Hey, everybody!" Gathering my composure, I said with as loud a voice as I could without screaming, "Basically, once you go to the second level, you have to get in a line to give your information to get on a plane. Once you get out of the first line, which is a mile long, you have to get in a second line, which is even longer. That puts you on a plane to somewhere in Texas either San Antonio, Austin, Dallas or somewhere like that. If you fly out of here, you will probably end up on a military base under marshal law for no tellin' how long!"

As soon as I stopped talking, obviously out of breath, everybody started yelling out expletives and complaints.

"Are you kidding me?"

"This is bullshit! I'm not gettin' on no plane!"

"Hell with that! What the ...?"

As I sat back down and listened to all the desperation and frustration, I looked forward and saw a news camera pointing in our direction, filming all the commotion. When the cameraman turned, I could see it was CNN News. The reporter was starting to talk to people and he would occasionally look back toward the camera. They were documenting this historic event. Historic, sad, and deplorable.

My phone vibrated in my pocket. Grabbing it, I looked at the screen and it read, "WHERE R U? WHAT IS GOING ON? TEXT ME OR CALL ME. MISS U. LORA."

I sent a message saying, "AT AIRPORT. IT' S CRAZY HERE. MAY HAVE TO CATCH PLANE TO TEXAS. MISS U 2. WILL TRY TO CALL. GAV." I pressed the send button and got the confirmation it was sent.

Turning toward my dad and Donna, I said, "I'm going to walk across Airline Highway toward my house to see how bad it is. We're (my dad and I) not getting on a plane unless we have no choice. I don't live too far from here, so I should be back in a couple of hours.

Dad, stay here, don't wander off anywhere!"

I leaned over to Donna and whispered in her ear, "Please keep an eye on him." She winked at me and nodded her head in acknowledgement.

Disconcerted, my dad said, "I'm not gonna wander anywhere, Son."

Donna caught me, "Hey Gavin, my son doesn't live too far from here. About a mile. Go by his house and see if they're there. He said he wasn't leaving for the storm." I walked back over to her and gave her a piece of paper out of my wallet and told her to write the address and phone number down, just in case the phone worked.

After getting the information, I told them I'd see them in a couple of hours, and I was off. It was after 4 p.m. now and still hot as could be. It didn't take five minutes of walking before I was covered in sweat. As I approached the Hilton Hotel across the highway from the airport, I could see there were all kinds of police and military personal walking in and out of the front door and was stopped by some sort of law officer. I didn't recognize his uniform, but he was obviously not going to let me in. Approaching him I said, "Hi, how ya doin'?"

He was a middle-aged white man who looked as tired as everyone else. He looked at me for a second or two and said, "Can I help you?"

Trying to be optimistic, I said, "I hope so. I just got evacuated from downtown to the airport and after asking around for a little while, I was told the only way out of the city was to get on a plane to Texas." I paused for a second and said, "I only live a couple of miles from here and wanted to go look at my house to see if it is livable."

Eyeing me up for a few seconds the man said, "You could try, but there are military road blocks set up all over the area. I doubt they will let you through, but you could try."

Pointing left and behind me, I asked, "How far down is the first road block?"

"Half a mile or so, I guess."

"All right, sir. Thanks for the info."

As I walked away, he said, "Wait a minute! There's another roadblock in the opposite direction about three miles down. I think if you can get someone to come get you they will let them through, providing proof they are here to get you."

Lora was in Texas. It would take at least eight hours for her to get me.

"Thanks again for the info, see ya later!"

"Good luck!"

I decided to walk toward the checkpoint in the direction of my house. It was closer to a mile than half a mile. At least it felt longer.

Nearing Williams Boulevard at Airline Highway, I saw two Hummer-looking vehicles with a few young National Guardsmen standing with guns directing various vehicles. There were also some state police in the area. I slowly walked up to one of those guys and asked, "Hi, how are you doing? I live (pointing to my left) a couple of miles from here. I just got evacuated from downtown and wanted to go see if my house is — "

Before I could finish my sentence he interrupted, "No, sorry. The area is on lock-down, and curfew will be starting soon. We're under Marshal Law!" I didn't even get to ask him anything else, as he just walked away from me. Aggravated, I walked off back toward the airport as the sun beat down on my sweaty, overheated body.

I started to feel as if my head was going to explode. I was getting very upset, anxious, overheated, and pissed off all at the same time. I started talking to myself, probably looking like a schizophrenic or something. A million thoughts collided in my mind. All of a sudden, I broke into an all-out sprint.

The next thing I know, I was leaning over trying to catch my breath. *What the hell am I doing?*

It took me about 20 minutes to get back to our spot.

Donna said, "Damn, that was quick!"

I'm sure I looked frustrated as I responded with, "They wouldn't let me go to my damn house! This is bullshit!"

Not even 30 seconds later I got a call that changed everything. Startled, I answered and was overjoyed to learn it was my friend, Corey. He lives in Bayou Gauche, which is south of New Orleans about 30 miles from downtown and about 20 to 30 minutes from the airport. With his subtle Cajun accent, he said, "Hey bra', you alive?"

With a surge of adrenaline I said, "Dude, I'm alive! I'm at the New Orleans airport. I just got here a couple hours ago, and it's fuckin' crazy here. Where are you?"

"I'm at home. We just got back earlier today from Shreveport.

Man, I saw the news and they showed your work and said there were riots and hostages and shit like dat!" "Corey, listen! You gotta come get us from the airport!

It's …"

"Who's us? Lora ain't with ya is she?"

"No, no! Me and my dad! His stubborn ass wouldn't leave so I got him to come down and stay with me at work. Big mistake."

I don't know exactly how he responded because as I was talking to him my phone started to beep and I saw it was from Lora's number. "Hey Corey, Hang on a second. Lora is trying to call me. If we get disconnected, call me back or text message me all right?"

Before I could hear his response, I clicked over and said, "Hey baby, am I glad to hear your voice!"

I could hear her starting to cry. "Are you okay?"

"Yes, Sweetie, I was just on the phone with Corey when you called. It was the first time my phone worked in a while. Did you get my text message?"

"Yeah, baby. I want to come get you, but they don't want me to!"

Stunned to hear her say that, I asked, "What? Who doesn't want you to?"

"Everybody. My family, your cousins ..."

Confused, I said, "My cousins? Who?"

"Scott and Craig. Baby, listen. It's crazy all over the state! The news is reporting people are stealing cars and when they run out of gas they are ramming other people's cars and stealing them! They're also saying gas is hard to get. Scott and Craig are worried something like that could happen to me."

I listened to her and couldn't believe what I was hearing. It was anarchy. Exasperated, I said, "They're tellin' us we have to get on a plane and go to Texas to military bases, and I'm not doin' that! Besides, my dad is out of his medicine ... I ... j -j-just ... damn ... shit man! Somebody's gotta come get us!"

I could hear her getting upset again saying, "Baby, what do you want me to do?"

She began to cry, and I started to feel bad. "Hey, hey, I'm sorry.

It's just insane down here. We gotta get outta here soon!"

Composing herself, she said, "Where's Corey ? Can he get y'all?"

"I don't know yet, I was in the middle of talking to him when you called." There was a second or two of silence and then I said, "I've been trying to find a way out of the city without getting on a plane. Everybody seems to be clueless as to what's going on. I tried to walk to the house, but was stopped and turned around by a military roadblock or whatever. I'm about to go and walk down to a checkpoint a few miles past the airport on Airline Highway toward Baton Rouge because someone told me they might let people through to pick up folks from the airport."

"Call me or text me when you find out."

"Hey Lora. Listen! Just in case my phone doesn't work ... keep in touch with me by text messaging and keep in touch with Corey.

Get a pen and write his number down!"

Hurriedly she said, "Hold on a minute!" I looked at my phone and saw the charge was dwindling down quickly. "All right, what's his number?"

I gave her the number and said to text message Corey if she needed to. Then, I lost the call.

You've gotta be kidding me.

I tried to call her back about five times with no success. I didn't realize it, but I had walked about a hundred yards away from our area. I turned around and went back to tell everybody, "Hey y'all, I'll be back in a little while. I'm gonna walk down to the checkpoint on Airline toward Baton Rouge to see if they're letting cars through to pick people up!"

Someone asked impatiently, "How far down is it?"

"About three miles, I think."

Someone else said, "Do your thang, G!" I waved back without even looking and away I went.

I decided to turn my phone off for a little while to conserve the battery. I was walking right in the direction of the setting sun, and it was blazing hot. You would think by now I would have been used to heat, but it was wearing me down.

About half a mile from the airport is an overpass bridge that goes over some railroad tracks, and once I was over the other side, I could see the checkpoint way down the road. It looked like an eternity, like a mirage, but in reality it was a couple of miles down the road. I walked another half a mile or so and a couple of cars passed me by. I decided to see if I could hitchhike (this would be a first) down to the checkpoint to conserve some energy.

About two minutes later, two African-American guys in a truck passed me by, then they stopped, pulled over, and started to back up. I jogged about 50 yards or so to meet them. "Hey guys, can I catch a ride down to that checkpoint there? I'm trying to get some information from them!"

"Yeah, no problem. Hop in the back there."

"Thanks!" I jumped in the back and sat on a spare tire. The breeze felt great. Simple things mean a lot when you're down to nothing. It was the first time I had cooled off in days, at least for a few minutes until we started to slow down near the checkpoint. As we came to a stop I stood up and jumped out and then walked up to the front to thank them.

One of the checkpoint guys pointed to us and said, "Wait a minute!" I stood there as this guy walked up to us.

I had renewed energy as I began my walk back to the airport. No matter if we had to sleep at the airport all weekend long, I now knew we did not have to get on a plane. Figuring this would be a good time to turn my phone back on, I did just that. I tried to call Lora a couple of times with no success. I then text messaged her saying, "THEY WILL LET U COME THROUGH CHECKPOINT TO GET US. CALL OR TEXT ME. GAV" After the "messaged sent" signal flashed, I tried to call Corey a few times with no success.

I frantically text-messaged him saying, "COREY TRY AND CALL ME BACK. THEY WILL LET U THROUGH THE CHECKPOINT ON AIRLINE HWY. TEXT ME IF U CANT CALL ME. GAV."

I decided just to walk back. I didn't want anyone to give me a ride, just in case they didn't have the necessary documents for their cars, and then I would get arrested or something stupid like that.

About five minutes later, my phone vibrated and the screen read, "DID U TALK 2 COREY? CAN HE PICK U UP? LORA"

Wiping the sweat from my brow, I sent back, "NOT YET. DID U TALK 2 HIM? I JUST SENT HIM A MESSAGE THAT HE COULD GET THROUGH CKPOINT."

I noticed I was walking faster than before, and by the time I sent the second message I had walked quite a bit closer to the airport. I was completely covered in sweat as the sun continued beating down on my back and head. I looked and saw a truck turned over and a house with the roof half blown off.

The area between the checkpoint and the airport was mainly filled with commercial businesses. It seemed like most of them sustained some sort of damage with blown out signs, torn off roofs, broken windows, and debris everywhere.

My phone rang and Lora's number flashed on the screen.

"Hello! Hello? Can you hear me?"

"Bay ...bee ...?" Then "CALL LOST."

I tried to call back with no luck. I then tried Corey with no luck. I was starting to get desperate. How the hell can the phone work a couple of miles away under a concrete and metal down ramp with hundreds of people using their phones, but it won't work out here in the wide open with no other phone in use? And at the worst time!

About 30 minutes later, I was nearing the airport, and there was a half-destroyed gas station on the right before the overpass bridge I had crossed before. About a 100 feet off, a woman pulling a suitcase behind her was walking toward me. When I got closer I could see she was wearing green nursing scrubs. She waved to me to come over as she walked toward the door of the beat-up gas station. Once I got close to her, she said, "Is this place open?"

It was obvious to me it wasn't, but I didn't want to be rude.

"No, I don't think so. Do you work at OPCSO (Orleans Parish Criminal Sheriff's Office)?"

"Why yes. Do you?"

"Yep, on HOD-10," I said, sticking my hand out and introducing myself. She did as well, but I don't remember her name.

She said she worked at CCC, which is the building across from HOD. She then said, "You're not going to Baton Rouge, are you?"

Pointing behind me, I said, "No, I just walked down to a check-point a few miles down the road, and they said that if you can get someone to pick you up, they will let them through to the airport.

Most of my family is in Texas, so I don't know when I'll get outta here, but I'm not getting in any of the lines or flying on any plane."

"Me neither, I'm gonna try and catch a ride to Baton Rouge, I guess."

Thinking about what Lora said, about the people stealing cars and ramming into other cars, I decided to warn her about what was going on the roads. She didn't seem too concerned. I looked around for a second or two and said, "Well, good luck. It was nice to meet you."

"You too."

As I got about a quarter mile away from the front exit of the airport, I could see a big jumbo cargo-looking plane take off in the distance. The closer I got to the front of the airport I saw people scattered everywhere. Groups of people sat in the grass, under trees, by the side of the road, and walking in every direction. There were thousands of people all over the place as I neared the entrance. I could hear the occasional person or group of people saying, "I ain't gettin' on no plane!" "We gotta get on a plane; we got nowhere to go!"

"I'll walk outta this mutha' fucka' before I get on a plane!"

"Are you crazy — you stupid!?"

It was amazing to hear the different people arguing about what to do. It was like a mass mental breakdown.

Approaching my dad and the others, I noticed most of the civilians and workers from the HOD building were sitting or standing from the end of the down ramp all the way to our area under the down ramp and beyond. I wasn't sure if people knew it or not, so I told a few people if they could get a ride out of here, or get someone to pick them up, they could. I was immediately bombarded with questions.

"Where did ya hear that, G?"

"Are you sure? You gotta ride or somethin'?" and other questions like that.

It had been a few hours now, and there was still a lot of uncertainty as to what was going on. The sun was again starting to set exquisitely in the distance. Just about everybody with a cell phone was trying to make calls, borrowing each other's phones or trying to send text messages. I sat down next to my dad and tried to get comfortable on the concrete.

Just as I leaned back, I felt something biting my lower right leg. Sitting up and slapping my leg, I saw a little bit of blood on my fingers. There were the remnants of a squashed mosquito. I said, "Great. With everything else going on we're gonna catch West Nile virus sitting here waiting to get outta here!"

My dad sat up and said, "What did you say?"

"Have you been getting bitten while I was gone?"

Looking a little confused he said, "Bitten by what?"

Trying not to look concerned I said, "I just killed a mosquito on my leg, and I hadn't noticed any before now." "I don't think so, Son, but I don't know."

Over the past few years in Southwestern Louisiana and, for that matter, the Southern United States, there have been quite a few deaths from the West Nile virus. Most deaths have affected older people and, as you might imagine, if I was getting bitten by mosquitoes, my dad was probably getting bitten too. The airport is located on the Jefferson Parish and Saint Charles Parish line and is surrounded by marshland to the west, with Lake Pontchartrain to the north. There are also low-lying areas around the airport that are perfect breeding grounds for mosquitoes.

Just as I was thinking of this, I saw my dad slap his right arm. He looked at his hand and had a tiny bit of blood and a smashed mosquito thrashing about. "I guess they are biting me."

"This is just great; we gotta get the hell out of here!"

In my mounting frustration, I stood up and walked around for a minute or two, slowly walking toward the center of the down-ramp and my cell phone miraculously rang.

It was Corey.

I didn't even give him a chance to say anything. "Dude, you gotta come get us ! Please!"

"Gav, I'm waitin' for my dad to come back with his truck."

"Hey man, I walked down to a checkpoint on Airline Highway between the airport and the I-310 exit (west of the city), and they said they would let people through to pick people up at the airport. Can you get us tonight?"

"I think so bra'. How bad is it?"

"Unbearable! Now the mosquitoes are starting to bite us! I don't wanna get West Nile out here. I definitely don't want my dad to catch it either — it could kill him."

"Hey, do I need to bring my gun or what? The news has been showin' some crazy shit."

"Corey! Bring whatever you want. I would suggest you bring your gun permit if you have one, and your driver's license."

I didn't realize it, but I must have started pacing, and as soon as I walked from underneath the down-ramp the call dropped.

"Corey! Corey!" Looking down at my phone it showed "CALL ENDED" and how long the call had lasted; not long enough.

These damn phones. I looked up and realized both times I lost the call I was not underneath the down ramp. I went back under the ramp and called Corey back. It took three tries, but I was finally able to get through.

"Corey? Can you hear me?"

"Hey, we got Lora on Darlene's (Corey's wife) phone. We're gonna try and come get ya'll."

"Hey, Corey, the entrance to the airport is blocked by police and the military. We're probably gonna have to walk out to the front and meet you somewhere."

"Where at?"

I thought about it for a second or two and then said, "There's a Denny's right across the street from the main exit, but the sign is halfway destroyed from the storm. What time do you have now?"

"About 7:30p.m .... Wait, hold on a second ... Darlene is talkin' to Lora."

As I waited for the relay message from Lora to Darlene to Corey and then to me, I walked over to my dad, smiled, and said enthusiastically, "I think we may get outta here tonight some time."

My dad looked up at me and said, "I don't feel like going anywhere, Son. I'm exhausted. Let's just stay right here tonight and go home tomorrow."

Almost dropping my phone I said, "What? Are you kidding? If Corey can come and get us tonight we're gettin' the hell outta here, that's for sure."

Before my dad could respond, Corey said, "I'm gonna get my gun and stuff together and come and get ya'll."

Pumping my fist in the air with excitement I said, "Man, I can't thank you enough. What did Lora say?"

"She was cryin' I think. She wants to come and git ya'll, but your family and hers won't let her leave. Too dangerous on the road or some shit like dat!"

"Yeah, I heard there's all kinds of wild stuff happening on the roads. Before I forget, take my dad's cell phone number down because my battery is gettin' low and his has a little more juice than mine."

"Hold on. Let me git a pen and paper."

As I waited, I couldn't help but smile a little, but the smile quickly left my face as I slapped my neck, killing another damn mosquito. I could see I was on my way to a blood transfusion at that rate. "All right, Gav, give me the number." I did and asked, "When do you think you'll be leavin'?"

"Within an hour or so. Hey, we don't have no power, just so you know. My parents have an RV that's runnin' off a generator, but they're stayin' in it. Y'all will have to stay at my house."

"I don't care if I gotta sleep in the garage. After where we've been, it doesn't matter."

Laughing a bit, he said, "Okay bra'."

"Corey, listen. I'll keep both phones on so call me when you're getting close because we're gonna have to walk from the main building out to Airline Highway to meet you." "Okay Gav, I'll see you soon — hopefully!"

"Great. Thanks. Bye."

After hanging up the phone, I sat back down next to my dad, saying, "Why in the hell would you want to stay here and get eaten up by mosquitoes? Lyin' on the concrete when we can go to somebody's house and you could lie on a couch and not risk getting the West Nile virus? In case you haven't noticed, we're a buffet for the mosquitoes right now!"

"I'm just tired; I don't feel like moving." He was fading fast.

"Well, Dad, it's too late. Corey is supposed to be on his way to get us."

"Who?"

He didn't have a clue who I was talking about. "My friend Corey. Remember I used to work for his dad about five years ago?

They live out in the country away from all this madness."

My phone rang, and it was Lora. I could hardly hear her, "Hey, is Corey coming to get you?"

"He's gonna try. I hope they'll let him through the road block."

"I love you Gavin! I miss you like crazy. You know that, right?"

Holding back tears I said, "I love you too! Stay by the phone and if Corey can get me tonight, I'll call you to let you know."

She said, "How's your dad?"

Walking away from him so he couldn't hear anything I said, "I don't know. Mentally, I'm not sure how he's coping. He keeps saying somethin' about going home. I've explained to him a thousand times his house may not be there."

"Don't be impatient with him! You know how you are."

"I'm tryin, but it's hard. What's even worse is the mosquitoes are startin' to eat us up, especially me. He says he doesn't feel them much, but I don't know how he doesn't feel them. He's sayin' he's too tired to move anywhere tonight, but I'll drag him kickin' and screamin' if I have too."

"Listen, baby, just talk to him calmly. Do you want me to talk to him?"

"Nah. Thanks, baby ... I got it. I hope to see you soon. If Corey can't get me tonight, I'm just gonna sleep here and try again tomorrow, but I'm not getting on any plane."

"If Corey can't get you, hopefully things in the next day or two will improve enough that I can come and get y'all."

"Honestly, baby, I think I might try to walk past the roadblock somewhere so Corey can get us. Either way, we gotta get away from the airport, because it's only gonna get worse. Well, sweetie, my battery is getting low. Hey, do you have my dad's cell number?"

"I don't think so — give it to me!"

I walked back over by my dad and I gave her his number.

Sitting down next to him, I said, "Lora says hi ... if we get to Corey's house soon, she will work on picking us up soon!"

I could hear Lora say, "Oohh! That sounded good. Maybe he'll like that."

My dad turned to me and said, "Well, if Lora can do that, then I guess we better get to whoever's house we're going to."

With some hopefulness for my dad, I said to Lora, "I'll talk to you later baby ... love you!"

"Love you too, Gavin, bye!"

After hanging up, I grabbed a water bottle out of my bag and chugged it down. Exhausted and restless at the same time, I got up and walked over to the mobile medical unit to have a look. It was dark by now and the sounds of helicopters, the roaring of generators, and people talking and moving around like ants filled the moment. The airport's electricity must have been running on generators because there were only a few main halogen lights shining through the blackness of the night. I decided to go to the second level and take one more look to see how bad it was. As I made my way up the stairs, I could hear the hustle and bustle of people shouting and ranting. When I got to the top level, there was still a mass of people everywhere. I didn't even bother going any farther. As I turned around, I saw a group of people coming up the stairs with all their bags and belongings. "Y'all goin' to get in those lines?"

A couple of them said, "Yeah, we ain't got no choice. We got nowhere to go."

Walking back down the stairs, I prayed we could get out of there that night. Not even five seconds after walking outside, I had mosquitoes all over me. I was waving my arms around, swatting bugs and looking like a crazy person. I grabbed my phone to see what time it was: 8:46 p.m. I saw two men in a fistfight as four or five law enforcement officials ran to break it up. There were people lying all over the ground trying to get settled for the night. It seemed as if some people were going to fly out as soon as possible, and others were resigned to stay where they were until most people were gone.

I could see my dad swatting his neck along with a few of the other people sitting near us. "Mosquitoes bad, huh, Dad? You still want to stay here tonight?"

"All right, Son, you made your point. Where are we going again?"

"Hopefully, my friend Corey, who lives about 20 miles or so from here, can get through the police checkpoint and pick us up. Hopefully."

"Yeah, hopefully. I've heard that before."

I had to bite my tongue once again. I was doing the best I could, and he didn't seem to appreciate it. I still wasn't sure he really knew the magnitude of what was going on. We'd gone from one serious threat to another all week.

Time crept by. With every swat and scratch of the mosquitoes, I was convinced one of us would end up sick. We had made it this far, and now we had to deal with this threat. I was more worried about my dad than myself, so I grabbed one of my shirts and fanned him. This served as a three-fold purpose: it kept me moving, hopefully keeping the mosquitoes off and it did the same for him; and it also gave him a breeze to keep him cool. I could see he appreciated it, but he didn't say anything. He forced a grin occasionally while shifting around trying to get comfortable.

The majority of people on the first level were under the downramp area because the main source of light was under there. Some people had dogs on leashes lying next to them. I would also sometimes see a dog wandering around without a leash. I began to wonder if some people just abandoned their pets or were unable to bring them on the departing planes. I also wondered where my mom was and if she was all right. From time to time I grabbed my phone to make sure I didn't miss a call or text message because sometimes, before the storm, my phone wouldn't ring or I would get a voicemail from the day before.

About 10 minutes later, I got a text message paging me to a phone number I didn't recognize. It had a "708" area code.

Where the hell is that? I leaned over and told my dad, "I'll be right back, I've gotta make a phone call."

"Who are ya calling, Son?"

"I'm not sure, Dad. This number popped up on my phone, and I have no clue who it is. I don't recognize the number." I put down my shirt and walked behind where we were to a spot that was a little less noisy, but I made sure to stay under the down-ramp. I dialed the number a couple times without it going through, of course. On the third try it started to ring, but the tone was very low. After about three rings, a female voice answered, but I didn't recognize the voice.

"Gavin...?"

"Hello ... who is it? I can barely hear you."

"Gavin, it's your mother!"

A little stunned to hear her voice I said, "Mom! Is that you, Mom?"

"Yes! Yes ... can you hear me?"

"Barely! Where are you?"

"I'm in Chicago at your Aunt Leslie's house. Where are you?"

"Dad and I just got evacuated to the airport a few hours ago from downtown, from work."

She must have sensed the desperation in my voice, "Son, are you all right?"

"It's been unbearably crazy the last five days. I don't know where we're goin' to end up. There's a slim chance I could end up in Texas somewhere on a military base under Marshal Law for weeks. I don't know. Dad is out of his medicine and keeps asking me when we're going home. It's chaos everywhere!"

"Did you say a military base in Texas?"

"Possibly. I'm trying to get my friend Corey to come and get us, but I don't know if he will be able to get through the roadblock."

There were a few seconds of silence before she said, "Did you say a roadblock? You're breaking up ..."

"Yes! There are military and police all over the place."

"You said your father is with you? Is he all right?"

"We've been through one hell of an ordeal, but he seems all right — physically, but I'm not sure mentally. You know how he is."

With a motherly concern in her voice, she said, "I love you, Son. Hang in there. Your father needs you. Be strong! I'll pray for the both of you."

"Mom, I have to save the battery on my phone, but I'm glad to hear your voice. Oh, before I forget, how's Alex (my half-brother)? Is he all right? Have you spoken to him?"

With a slight crack in her voice she said, "Not yet, but knowing Doc (Alex's father), they probably evacuated. I haven't been able to get through to his cell phone, but I'll keep trying."

"Well, I'm glad you're all right, Mom, and I'll call you as soon as I end up wherever I end up."

"I love you Gavin and I'm gonna pray for you and your father's safety!"

"Me too. Love you. Bye."

After hanging up with my mom, I felt a huge sense of relief that she was all right, and I wondered if Alex was too. My gut told me he was alive, but I just didn't know. I sat back down next to my half-asleep dad. I swatted his right arm below his elbow, killing another mosquito.

Please God, let us get out of here tonight, please! Please, don't let anything happen to my dad!

Putting my head between my legs, I strained to hold back tears. Composing myself, I grabbed the shirt on top of my bag and started to fan my dad again. It was nighttime now and once again, the stars covered the sky. The people scattered on the ground level of the airport were starting to settle in to their areas, resigned to the fact they were going to be there for the night, if not longer. Everybody had some piece of cardboard or paper and fanned himself or herself to try and cool off.

Occasionally, vehicles drove by, but they were few and far between. I didn't know if that meant they were only letting a few cars past the checkpoint or if it took a long time for each car to pass through it.

I was gazing in the general area of the exit when my phone vibrated again. The message read, "IN LINE AT CHECKPOINT. LINE IS LONG. WILL CALL IF WE GET THRU. COREY." I looked at the time, and it was about 9:30.

I decided not to say anything to my dad, knowing he wouldn't have anything positive to say. Feeling ever so close to getting to some sort of safety, I continued to fan my dad relentlessly. I only felt a few bites. I did my best to keep the mosquitoes off of my dad.

It looked like a war zone. Just about everybody was sitting or lying on the ground, half asleep or slumped over. Obviously, the past four or five days had taken their toll. I was one of the few people standing, and to be honest, I didn't know how.

It was creeping upon 10:30. The charge on my phone was waning, and I was fearful it would go dead before we got out of there. Checking my dad's phone, I saw that his was about half-charged, but it didn't seem to be working that well. My dad was dozing, periodically wiping and scratching his face and irregularly snoring. I was beginning to think Corey wouldn't be able to get through to rescue us.

Not a minute later, my phone rang. It was him. "Hey dude, the line is barely moving ... I'm gonna try to go down River Road and cut through that way."

"Yeah, okay. Whatever you can do. I'll be waitin' for your call."

"All right, bra'... later."

"Later."

It was so close I could almost taste it. Freedom and safety, that is.

Well, not really, but I was really feeling better. At least he was trying to get to us. I knew he would do whatever he could to make it happen. All I could do was fan the old man and keep my fingers crossed Corey would get here without getting arrested or something.

For the next 45 minutes, I tried to keep my dad cool and reflected on the past few days. It was amazing to think about how much had changed in such a short time. I really liked my job and where we lived, and now everything had changed. I didn't realize it, but I was sitting down next to my dad drinking a bottle of water, and I didn't even remember getting the water out of my bag.

Finally it came. The call!

It was almost 11:30 on Friday night, September 2. Five days after Katrina came ashore in New Orleans, eight days after it hit southern Florida: "Hey Gavin, we're in front of the Denny's. Get your ass up here as fast as you can, before I shoot one of these mother fuckers walkin' around my truck!"

"All right, all right! Give me about 10 minutes. We have to walk from the main area to the exit. We're comin' right now!"

"Hurry up!"

I didn't even say "bye" as I ended the call. "Dad, wake up. We're leavin'!"

Disoriented he said, "I'm too tired to go anywhere."

"What? Get your ass up now! Corey is waiting for us. Get up! Get up!"

"All right ... all right, Son. Hang on a minute."

As I pulled up the bag he was lying on, Nurse Donna saw me gathering my stuff together and said, "Where the hell are you going?"

"We're outta here baby! I gotta get him away from these mosquitoes. My friend just called and said he is front of the Denny's waitin' for us."

"Well, Gavin, take care and good luck."

Leaning over and giving her a hug I said, "You too! I'll see ya ... good luck to y'all too!"

Grabbing both bags and putting one on each shoulder, I said goodbye to those around me. As we began to walk toward the exit, I didn't realize how many people I would see between the down ramp and the exit, but I said goodbye what seemed like a hundred times. It was really strange, but I felt like a chapter in my life was ending, and I realized I probably wouldn't see many of those people ever again.

My dad was trying to walk as fast as he could, swerving back and forth, and stumbling a couple of times. As we passed the bottom of the down-ramp, it was so dark I could hardly see. I had to stop a couple times to wait for my dad to catch up and to rest my shoulders from the weight of the bags.

"I'm walking as fast as I can, Son ... I can't see too good in the dark."

"I didn't say anything, Pops. Take your time."

Approaching the exit, I could see what looked like

Corey's truck parked across the highway on the edge of the Denny's parking lot. Everything felt like it was in slow motion as we neared the truck.

Police or military personnel (it was so dark I couldn't tell) were directing traffic and telling people to get off the road. I waved one over to me and said, "That's my ride over there (pointing about 50yards away)."

"All right, hurry up and get across the street!"

I hooked my dad's left arm with my right as I grabbed my phone, balancing both bags on each shoulder. I called Corey as we walked across the street. "Dad, it looks like we made it out of the city alive!"

"What's that? Oh, yeah, I guess so ... where are we going again?"

"To Corey's house. Don't worry about it ... it'll be better than the airport, I promise."

Corey must have seen us coming across the street because he got out of his truck. "Hey bra', y'all get in on my side ... throw your bags in the back." As I threw my bags in the back, Corey helped my dad get into the back cab of the truck. Corey's wife, Darlene, was sitting in the front passenger's seat looking a little paranoid.

I saw Corey's handgun sitting on the center console. "You brought some firepower with you, I see."

Closing the door he said, "Dude, I was sure I was goin' to have to shoot somebody about five minutes ago. They had all kinds of sonsabitches walkin' around my truck!"

His wife said, "Yeah. It's so dark. We thought somebody was gonna try and carjack us!"

They both turned to my dad and said, "How ya doin?"

Not really sure who they were he said, "Oh, I don't know, okay, I guess."

I could see he was a little unsure, so I said, "Dad, you remember Corey. I used to work for his dad a few years ago, and this is his wife Darlene."

It took him a few seconds, but then he said, "Oh yeah, 'hi'

Corey and what's your name again, Sweetheart?"

Smiling at me, she answered, "Darlene."

"Nice to meet you."

As he sat back, I said, "Hey y'all, thanks for comin' to get us — I can't thank you enough. If y'all wouldn't have come we might have been shipped out on a plane to Texas somewhere or a military base. That might have been worse than everything we've been through already."

Corey turned the truck around and we drove about a mile and then took a turn and drove toward River Road (a road on each side of the Mississippi River that snakes around for many miles in both directions).

"Why are we going this way?" I asked.

Corey replied, "The line coming in was really bad so we cut through and down River Road, where some of those orange and white road blocks set up, but we went around 'em." Sure enough, there was a "Road Closed" sign blocking the road up ahead and we went right around it. We eventually got to the I-310 loop that went south towards Highway 90 (south of the city).

As we took the loop, there were no streetlights anywhere. It was like we were driving through outer space, with only our headlights to guide us. We made small talk with them for the next 15 minutes or so with my dad falling half asleep while we drove.

When we turned onto Bayou Gauche Road, Corey said, "Now, remember, we ain't got power at our house. My parents are staying in their RV, which is running off of a generator, and we'll be staying with them. During the day, y'all can hang out in there."

Making sure he knew how grateful I was, I said, "Hey man, don't even worry about that. We'll be fine. I'm just lookin' forward to taking a shower. I haven't had one in about six days!"

Laughing, Corey said, "Yeah, I can tell!"

I laughed and Darlene slapped Corey on the shoulder, "Oh, Corey!"

After another second or two of laughter, I blurted out,

"That's all right, Darlene. He's right!"

"Hey bra', you know it'll be a cold shower!"

"Man, I don't care if ice cubes come out of the shower head; I'm takin' a shower."

As we turned down his street, he asked us if we wanted something to eat. I kindly declined for my dad. I woke him up and told him, "We're here — let's go take a shower."

Corey grabbed his flashlight and led us inside. He and Darlene got us set up with pillows as I made a bed on the floor and made a bed on the couch for my dad. They had some water in an ice cooler and some snacks on the table for us. We thanked them again, and they left and went down the street to his parents' RV. We navigated to the bathroom by flashlight, and I got Dad in the shower. I held the light over the shower curtain so he could see what he was doing. After he was done, I jumped in and let the frigid water run over my head and body.

"Wow," I said out loud.

"Boy, you said it!" my dad chimed in.

"This sure beats sleeping outside on the concrete while getting eaten up by mosquitoes!"

"You're right, Son!"

Corey had left us some clean T -shirts and shorts to sleep in, since all of our stuff was dirty and smelly. As we lay down to sleep, there were a few minutes of silence. As I was falling asleep, my dad whispered, "I love you, Son... thanks for getting us out of the city."

I reached up from the floor and patted him on the back, holding back tears and said, "Love you too, Buddy. You know I'll always be here for you. Goodnight."

"Goodnight, Son."

Within a couple of minutes, he was gently snoring and I drifted off too.

We'd made it.

Chapter 16

After the Storm

The next morning when I woke up, it took me a moment or two to remember where I was. My dad was still sleep, or so I thought. I didn't hear him snoring, and I didn't hesitate to check to see if he was breathing. On cue, he let out a big snore as I was about to wake him up. Laughing to myself, I just let him sleep.

I got up and went out the back door to check out the surrounding and to reflect on the past week. *What a week it was!*

I took another cold shower, and my dad woke up about 9:30 or so, and like me, he didn't quite know where he was. Corey and Darlene came down from his parents' place and offered us some coffee and a hot breakfast. A smile came across my dad's face like I hadn't seen in quite a while. "Hell yeah!" he said, while he scrambled for his clothes and shoes.

For the rest of the day Corey's parents were out and about, and they let my dad and me stay in their motor home, where we had our first taste of real air-conditioning in over a week. It was glorious.

They also had a television, and we were able to catch up on what was going on and how the country was reacting to this national disaster. Since there was no electricity and the generators ran off of gas, they periodically turned off the generators to conserve energy. I noticed Corey's mom, Ms. Maxine, had some clothes hanging on a clothes line, and I asked her if I could wash our clothes since ours were all dirty.

Smirking slightly, she directed me to a plastic tub, liquid detergent, and a water hose and said, "Here's the washing machine!"

It was then that I got a glimpse of the old days, when the washing was done by hand and hung to dry. In order to get our clothes cleaner, I used the back of a shovel handle to churn the water and clothes. I was amazed to see the water turn a dark shade of gray. Who would have known in this day and age, clothes could get clean in by using a bucket?

It didn't take long for my dad to start asking, "When are we going home? I need to get my medication." I had to continue to explain to him what had really happened and there was no guarantee we had a home to go home to.

I was able to call Lora. She said she and my two cousins, Scott and Craig (from Paris and McKinney, Texas), were coming to get us on Monday afternoon — hopefully.

"They're in the process of getting gas cans and filling them up so we can leave early Monday morning ... you need to decide where we can get y'all. José (my sister-in-law's boyfriend) said he can get y'all from Corey's and bring y'all somewhere off I-10 to meet us."

Just when I thought I would have some down time, I was right back on the phone talking with my wife, José, and others trying to get us to Texas. I had charged my phone on Corey's parents' generator and was able to use it without worry it would die.

My Aunt Sandra lives in Paris and told Lora she had a place for us to stay and a little cottage for my dad to stay in while we got our plans together. At least we had a place to stay, but I was faced with the proposition of telling my dad we were on our way to Paris, Texas, to stay for a while and not home where he desperately wanted to be.

After finally getting off of the phone, we sat around most of that evening as I told them what the city looked like after the storm blew through and about our adventures in the aftermath. After a nice home-cooked dinner, our first in a week, we were down the street getting ready to sleep. Although it was quite hot, it was nothing compared to the stench-filled sweltering heat we were in for six days.

Most of Sunday was spent finalizing our plans to get to Texas. I decided to check on my condo after hearing on the news Jefferson Parish was opening up (under curfew) for residents who wanted to assess their property damage. After speaking to José, I made a decision to catch a ride with him on Monday morning to Kenner to see how bad it was.

Our entertainment for the day came courtesy of my dad. We were sitting by the Katrina-polluted pool in the backyard of Corey's parents' house. It was steamy hot, so we moved under the back patio into the shade. In south Louisiana, there are countless numbers of critters, and we have millions of "love bugs" (they mate for 24 hours and die) during the late summer. As we sat around and shot the breeze, my dad started swatting love bugs away from him. This was funny by itself. About five minutes later, he looked to his left and saw the wooden gate open. We watched him get up, mumble something, and walk over to the gate and close it. As he sat back down he announced to us,

"Maybe if we keep the gate closed, we can keep those damn bugs out!"

We all looked at each other, smiling and trying to hold back our laughter. He was serious, too. I realized he was so exhausted he had mentally slipped a little more. I hadn't been able to see him as much in recent years, but after spending that week with him up close, I concluded we were at the point in our lives I had been dreading for a long time.

You can't escape Father Time, and as much as my dad likes to think he's 50 years old, he's not. From then on, I would be keeping a close eye on him.

On Monday morning, I was on the phone again. Lora called and said they were on their way from Texas, and we decided to meet in LaPlace (a suburb further west from the airport) in the early afternoon. We agreed to stay in contact with each other periodically throughout the day. I then made arrangements with José to go into Kenner to see how bad the condo was.

Corey's wife gave me a ride to Corey's work, and he gave me a ride to LaPlace because he didn't want her to drive without him. I couldn't really blame him. That turned out to be a mistake. José and I agreed to meet in the Home Depot parking lot in LaPlace and then take Airline Highway into Kenner. This is about a 12- to 14-mile stretch of road and was the only main road into town, as the I -10 at LaPlace was closed to incoming traffic. Once we got to Home Depot and met José and his friend, reality struck.

There was a line of cars in both lanes bumper-to-bumper for as far as I could see leading into the city and back to the west toward Baton Rouge. I understood I would be unable to get into Kenner, assess the damage, and get back in time to meet Lora and my cousins.

Also, it would take extra time for them to get into LaPlace. We went back to Bayou Gauche and then to Raceland via Highway 90. As we made our way back, we had to go down River Road toward Baton Rouge, over the Sunshine Bridge and back to Bayou Gauche to pick up my dad. The next time I was able to speak to Lora, they were just passing through Baton Rouge, making great time. Unfortunately, I had to tell them to turn around and come back through Lafayette, going south through Houma down Highway 90 so we could meet them in Raceland somewhere.

We met at the Shell station on Highway 90 in Raceland. After we packed me, my dad, José's friend, his dog, and José into his Nissan Altima, I thanked Corey and his family for everything they had done for us. We said our goodbyes, and then we made our way to the gas station, which was about 15 miles from Corey's house.

Once we were dropped off at the Raceland Shell station, my dad and I sat in the mini-restaurant area. Before long, he was up and roaming around the store as I struck up a conversation with a guy who was sitting down to eat. Come to find out, the man owned some businesses about a half-mile from my home, and he described the scene to me. I'll spare the details, but from what he said, his places had substantial damage, and I could only assume mine did as well.

It was after 3 p.m., and my dad had purchased some clipon sunglasses and a bunch of junk food. As he stuffed his face, I got a call from my cousin Scott who said, "Is there anyway you can hitchhike from where you are down the road a few miles or so? We're at some sort of checkpoint, and there are a bunch of cars in front of us. It could take hours from here to get to y'all. I'll pay big money to anyone in there who'll give you guys a ride."

I told him I'd call him back in a couple of minutes as I stood up to start looking around to see who I could ask for a ride. The man I was talking to eventually agreed to give us a ride, but I had to convince him first, because it was in the opposite direction of town. He kept insisting that he just came through a roadblock and was sure I was telling him the wrong way.

Once I was able to convey to him we were going the other way, he finally realized he was turned around and said, "You're right — let's go!" I rounded up my dad, grabbed our stuff, and we got in this man's truck. I called Scott, told him we had a ride, that we were in a black truck and the guy who was bringing us would not go past the checkpoint.

"That's great, Gavin. We'll cut across the median and back up to y'all!"

As we approached the checkpoint, our side of the road was clear, with no one stopping and no one checking any cars. The other side had a few police units and, I guess, state policeman checking every car. Both lanes were full of cars as far as I could see, and I had no idea how far down Lora and my cousins were.

The man who drove us said, "This is as far as I'm gonna go fellas."

I called Scott back and told him to cut across the highway and we were on the side of the road in a new black Ford truck. Not even 10 seconds later, I could see a white Chevy Suburban about a mile down the road sharply cut across the grassy median and backing up down the shoulder toward us.

As we got out of the truck, I thanked the man for the ride, grabbed our bags, and put one on each shoulder. It didn't take them long to get to us and as they stopped and got out, I immediately made eye contact with Lora and we both let out a sigh of relief. I couldn't believe how thin her face looked; in just nine days she had lost a good deal of weight. I knew she was worrying, but I could clearly see how this ordeal took its toll on her. I shook hands and hugged both of my cousins and then hugged my wife as tightly as I could, both of us wordlessly shedding a few tears.

I could hear Scott thanking and offering the man who had given us a lift some money, but the man said, "No thanks, that's all right." Out of the corner of my eye , I saw my dad walking toward Scott and Craig, shaking their hands and letting out his own sigh of relief.

We eventually put our bags in the back of Scott's Suburban and drove off toward the setting sun.

This part of the journey finally ended in Paris, Texas at about midnight. After 10 hours, we finally got to the room at the Best Western where Lora and her family had been staying.

Finally! Whew!

A few days later, I rented a car and drove back to New Orleans to see how bad the damage was to my home. The drive was dream-like. I still couldn't believe everything that had happened. With all the gas shortage concerns, I stopped about seven or eight times before I got to the city limits. It was during this drive I made the decision to write a book.

For some reason, I felt I was supposed to be in it, and it was meant to be. Hopefully, things would work out. I first went to my dad's house to see how it fared. To my surprise, his place had minimal damage, and I was able to save his treasured instruments: a saxophone, clarinet, and a flute. After spending about three or four hours cleaning out his refrigerator and throwing out some stuff that got wet from a couple of leaks, I left and made the long drive to our house to assess the damage.

After navigating through the numerous military checkpoints, I arrived at our home. The damage was pretty bad. About three feet of water was pooled in the downstairs portion of the condo and a six- to eight-foot area of the ceiling in the master bedroom had caved in. I vividly remember looking around in shock, not knowing where to begin the clean-up process.

Navigating around all of our water-logged stuff, the smell was horrid. I could only assume with all of the flooding, some of the nasty-looking water from a nearby canal made its way into our house. The smell could have also been from the water just sitting in our house for a while; I really don't know. The back patio area looked like a bomb had gone off. The fence was gone and most of the plants and the vine trellis was destroyed. I really believe that a twister or something must have caused the ceiling in the bedroom to cave in and destroy the backyard. Mine is a corner unit and the building right behind had much less damage. I attempted to clean up the place for a few hours and punched holes in the sheetrock, (as advised by a neighbor), so the mold wouldn't spread as fast.

As the evening approached, I left and spent the night at Corey's house. I brought some of our salvageable pictures to his house. The video tape of my wedding was in the downstairs T.V. stand and had been completely submerged in water and still very wet. Corey suggested putting it in the refrigerator to get the condensation out, and to my surprise we later played the video and found it worked.

The next day, I went back to my dad's place to finish cleaning up, which was another six or seven hours of hot, hard work. Once I was finished with that, I drove back down the West Bank Expressway, taking a mental note of all the wind damage to countless businesses and homes. It was hard to look at so much devastation, but after what my father and I had gone through, it really didn't surprise me. I eventually made it back to my house, did some more cleaning, and drove back to Texas to be with Lora and the dogs.

The time away gave me a chance to get closer to my family. Being the youngest cousin on my father's side by quite a few years, I really never had the chance to be close to my cousins and my Aunt Sandra. My Aunt Sandra was married to my dad's brother, my Uncle Tommy, who died about 15 years ago. Although I didn't know it, his death really affected my dad quite a bit. During the time before and after I arrived in Texas, Scott and his mother were wonderful to Lora and her family. As a matter of fact, the whole city of Paris, Texas, was wonderful to them and all the other Louisiana evacuees who ended up there.

We stayed in Texas for almost a month. Lora eventually got a call to go back to work teaching at the school she was at before. On a whim, I called my supervisor at work and asked what was going to happen with my job. To my utter surprise, he said they were going to reopen the HOD building in midOctober. I asked him if they were going to bring anybody back and he said he would find out. A couple days later he called and asked if I could like to come back, and I jumped at the offer. There were over 70 nurses who worked at the jail before the storm and they only brought back 10 of us at first, which made me feel pretty good (and lucky). Besides, Lora and I really needed the health insurance to take our last try at the in- vitro process. I went back to work in mid-October and was able to see the mass destruction first hand. We eventually found out the eggs were moved soon after The Storm and we pray they will be alright so we can try one more time.

Of the numerous facilities within the jail system, only the HOD building, where my father and I were stranded, was salvageable to the point of re-opening the jail system for the city of New Orleans. I really had to see it to believe it. The first building I went into was the CCC building. There were breaches in many of the tier walls.

Those walls were made with cinder blocks and obviously were not made very well. I was told by one of the deputies that fire extinguishers were used by the inmates to knock holes in the walls in an attempt to escape the facility. Some did escape, including a man from St. Bernard parish who was in for murder. He got as far as Mississippi before he killed another man and was caught.

In all, I have heard estimates there was over $100 million dollars in damage to the entire parish penal system, and from what I saw, that could be fairly accurate. All the buildings sustained heavy flooding, and many of them were beyond repair. I don't know what the future will hold for the city of New Orleans, but I will be able to watch firsthand what the new New Orleans will begin to look like.

With everything that happened, I am still blessed my father was alive and we'd survived the ordeal of our lives together. I was not able to find out what happened to the lady who was holding up the sign. I can only hope that she made it out.

My little brother Alex made it out and would eventually go back to Waveland, Mississippi, to find where he lived was totally devastated. He stayed there for a while and eventually joined the Army and is currently in Iraq defending our country. He recently dodged death as he was in a Humvee hit by a roadside bomb. After sustaining second degree burns and an injured knee, he was able to cut loose a fellow trooper and get them to safety under enemy fire. God bless him.

I have been working at the facility ever since we came back to the city and have not seen J.W. since. I hope he is all right and getting the psychiatric treatment he so desperately needs.

Nurses Robert, Donna, Urban, Favis and a few others have come and gone since. As we were evacuating, there were many times when I didn't think I would see those people again. I am glad I did and have formed a closer bond with them because of what we went through.

The only person I heard about that had a major physical problem was Deputy Lee. I found out about three months later Deputy Lee ended up in Houston and had three surgeries on that toe to try and save it. Unfortunately, the surgeries were unsuccessful, and he ended up getting the toe and part of his foot amputated.

As I move forward in my life, I will always remember this experience and keep it near to my heart. I know I will share it with generations to come. While I didn't appreciate the circumstances while they were unfolding, the experience shaped who I am and the choices I will make for the rest of my life.

THE END

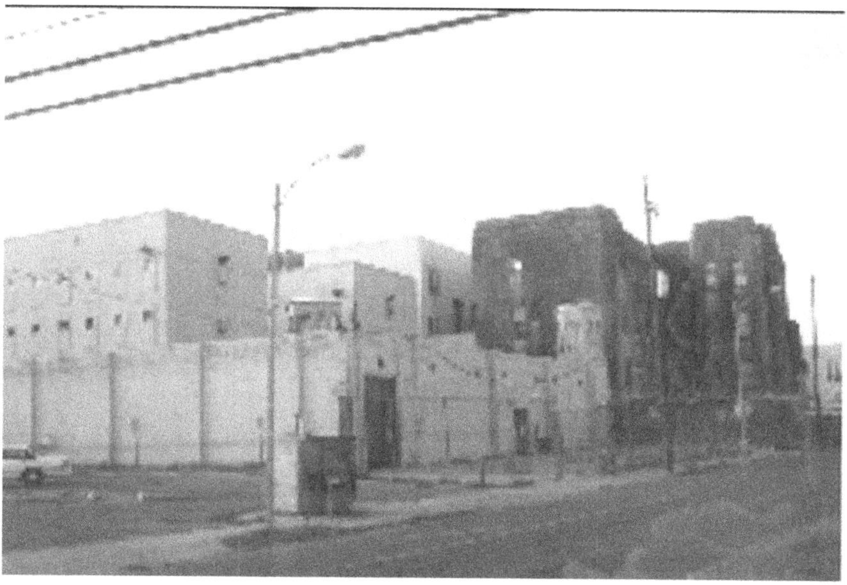

The back side of O.P.P. which is connected to the New Orleans District Courthouse on the corner of Tulane Avenue and Broad Street in New Orleans.

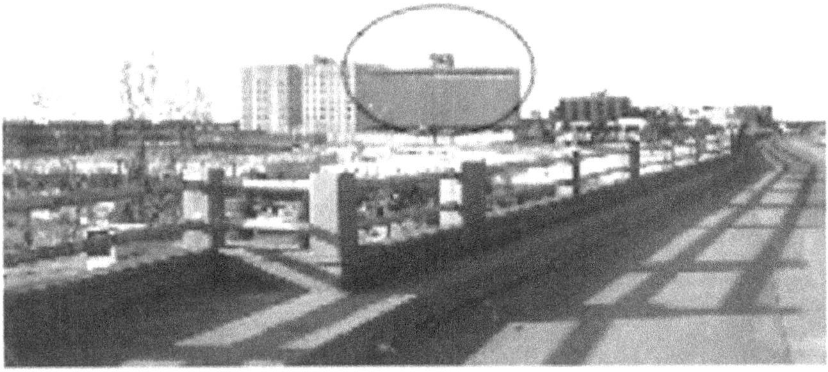

The center building is House of Detention as seen from the Broad St. bridge. The CCC building is to the left.

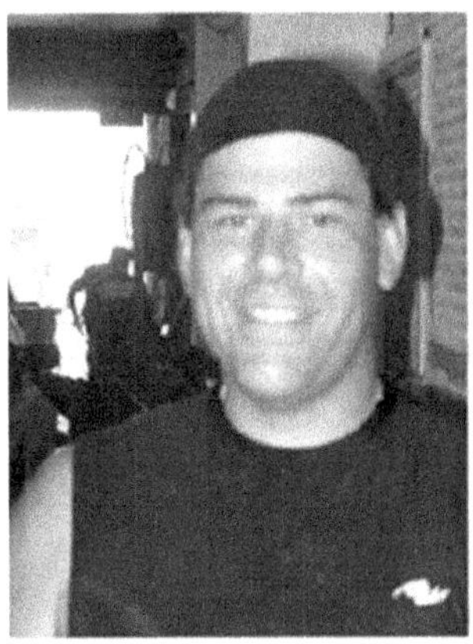

Nurse Robert Gates who has been with the Sheriff's office for over 15 years, mostly working at the House of Detention.

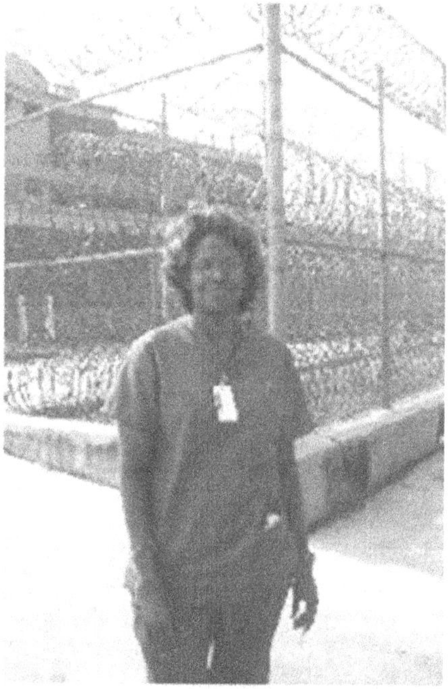

Nurse Favis, LPN, who worked at the Sheriff's office less than two years when Hurricane Katrina hit.

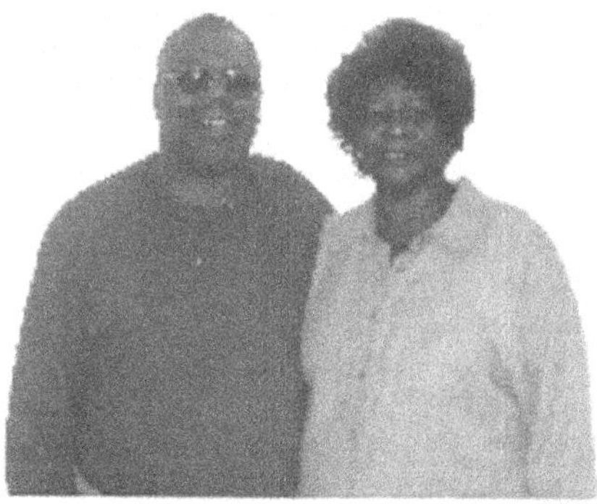

John and Nurse Donna Landry

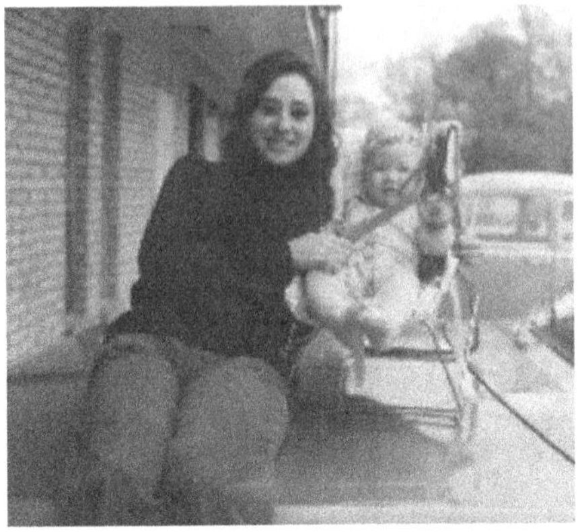

My mother, Roberta, with me, Gavin Johnson, as a baby.

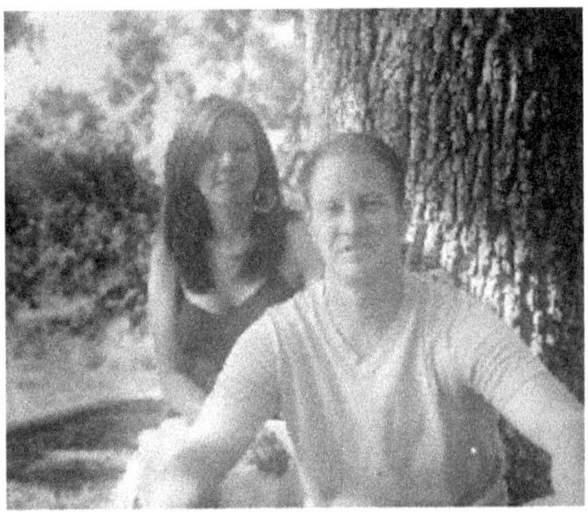

Lora and Gavin Johnson.

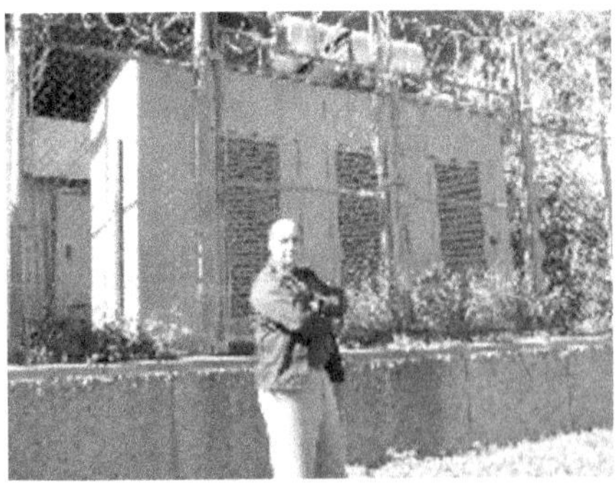

Dr. Marcus Dileo, whose heroic efforts saved many lives at Orleans Parish Prison in the aftermath of Katrina. He swam in contaminated waters to attend to others, with no regard for his own safety.

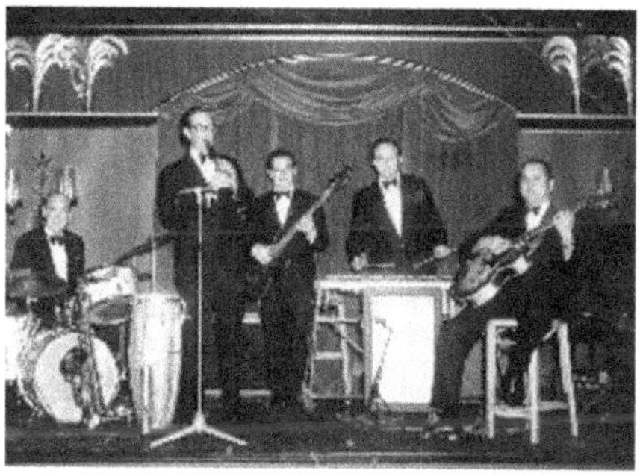

Liston Johnson, (playing clarinet) with his quintet in the good old days.

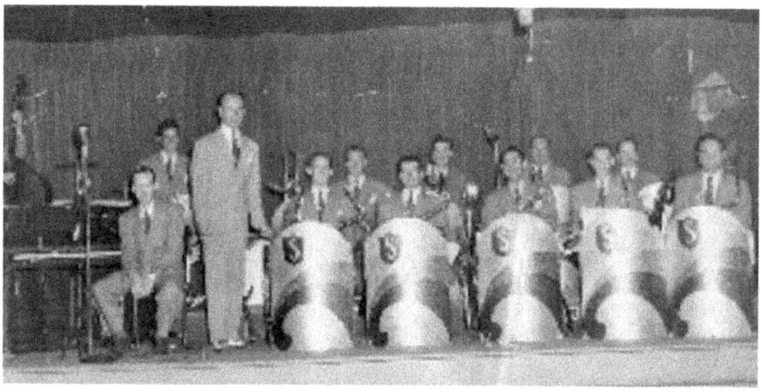

Liston Johnson, in the Gus Arnheim Band (immediate right of Gus), Los Angeles, 1942.

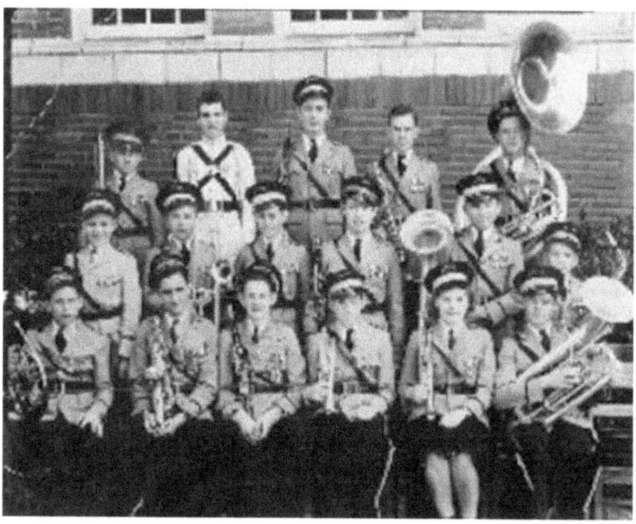

My father (third from left, front row) in a school band in his youth.

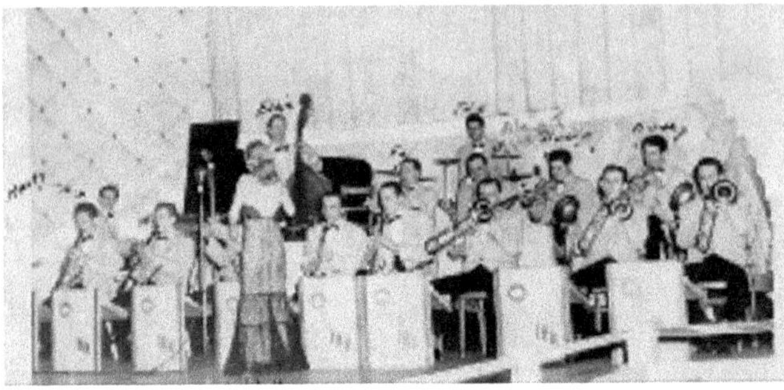

My father (far left on clarinet) in Ina Hutton Band, 1946. Al Hirt is in the back, top row.

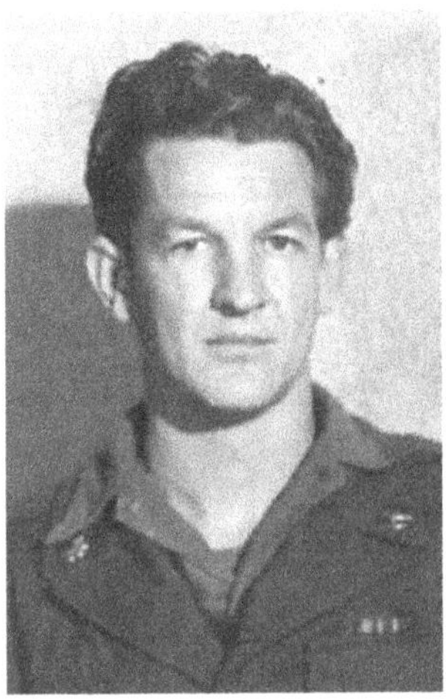

My father, Liston Johnson in Army uniform during World War II.

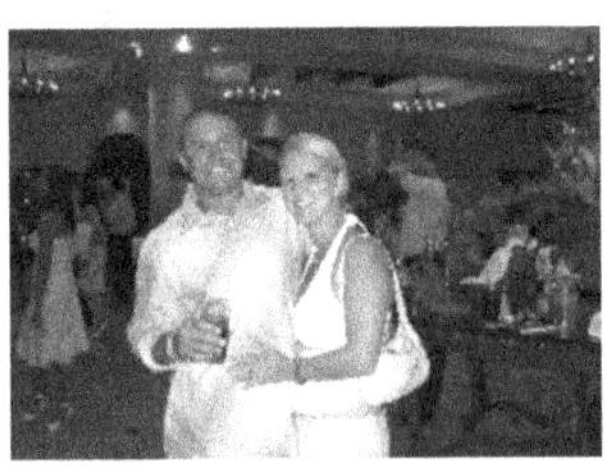

My friend Corey Dufrene with his wife Darlene. They drove in with a handgun for protection and rescued me and my father from the New Orleans airport. They took us to safety at his parents' house in Bayou Gauche.

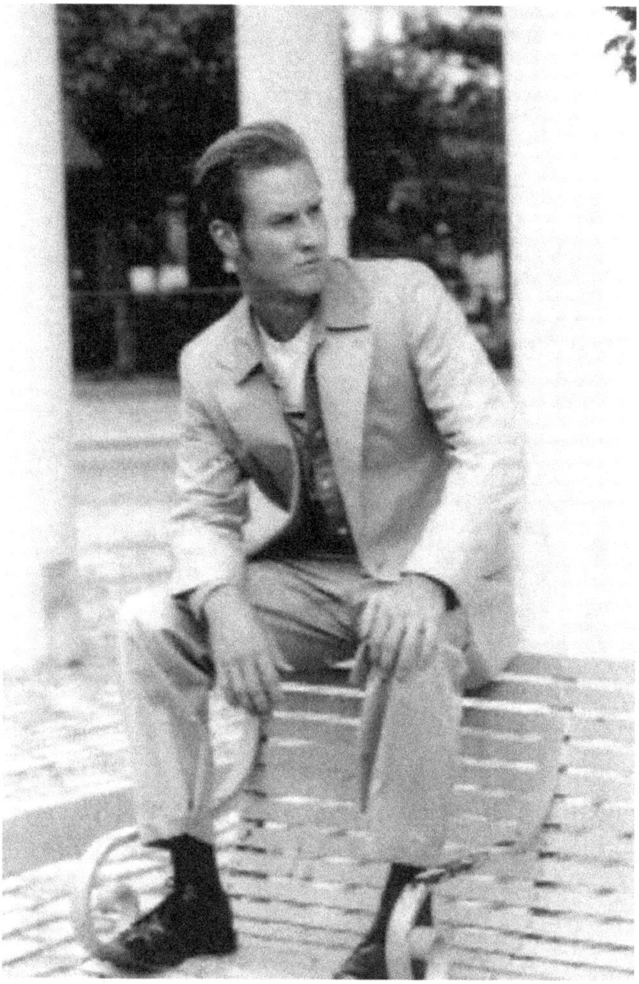

The author, Gavin S. Johnson, a native New Orleanian, is a psychiatric nurse who worked at Orleans Parish Prison's House of Detention when Hurricane Katrina hit. He rode out the storm and its aftermath at the jail facility with his 83-year-old father, Liston, before getting them both to safety.

Epilogue

Wow… What a journey! These past 20 years have flown by. Hard to believe I'm 53 years old. When I look in the mirror I don't love what I see lol, but I certainly don't feel 53. My dad passed away in 2014 at the age of 92 and lived a pretty good life. My brother Alex passed away suddenly at the age of 27, having completed 2 tours of duty in Iraq and was a decorated service member. Rest in peace my brother. Next, my 2 pugs passed away in 2015 and the beginning of 2016. My little girl pug was diagnosed with diabetes at age 5 for which I was told she would probably only live about a year as dogs are only type 1 diabetics. This didn't seem like it should be the case, so I did some investigating and experimenting and the results were quite amazing. It was quite expensive, but I was able to get insulin for her and after some trials and tribulations, I settled in on 10 units of long-lasting insulin 2 times a day and she lived to be 13 years old! The veterinarian was amazed and had never seen any of his animal patients live that long. Those 2 dogs were such a blessing, and I miss them every day. It's truly amazing the love you feel for a pet and how painful it is to lose one. Of course, I was very sad when my dad passed away but as we all know that is inevitable. The pain of losing a pet just feels a little different. It's got to be unconditional love that they give to you. No doubt God gave us animals to show us how to love unconditionally, but many of us struggle to do so. Will be one of the 1st questions I will be asking when I hit the afterlife!

Unfortunately, after the Hurricane, there was a steady decline in his health and a few situations where he must have had a guardian angel looking over him. In 2008 his car got stole right in in front of his house. This happened on a Friday night, and he called me the next morning saying his car was gone. Of course, I said "what do you mean your car is gone…"

"Son, I don't know… All I know is that my car isn't there…"

This set off an unbelievable chain of events that I couldn't have imagined. I left my house and drove to his house to investigate. Sure enough, the car was nowhere to be found so I called the cops to make a stolen car report and then called his insurance company. He immediately wanted to get another one or at least a rental but nothing was available until Sunday afternoon. I had to work that evening, so we made an appointment to get him a rental car at a place that was about 15 minutes from his apartment.

When we got there, the only car they had available was a metallic light blue PT cruiser and his eyes lit up when he saw it. Remember he was about 85 years old at this point and not the best driver for sure. We got the car and I followed him to a point where it was time for me to go to work and at the red light were we went our separate ways. I instructed him to go home, and he acknowledged me. When I got to work I called him but he didn't answer. No big deal so I thought. At about 10 pm I called his cell phone again and no answer. I was scheduled to get off at 11pm but I called my supervisor and let her know I had to leave and drove straight to my dad's house. To my surprise and angst, he was not home and all the lights were off. This was not normal. I went outside to see if I saw his new shiny rental car and I did not see it anywhere. I immediately got in my car and started driving around the area where he lived. It's on the west bank of New Orleans and not that big of an area. After driving around for about an hour or so, I decided to go to the Police Station and report him missing. I'm assuming he's joy riding but my gut tells me otherwise.

Upon telling the cop at the station the situation, he informed me that someone must be missing 24 hours before an official report can be done. I explained the situation to him again and how unusual it is for him to be out past dark and would he reconsider. He ended up talking to someone else and came back with some very disturbing news. Come to find out they found my dad's stolen car in a ditch full of bullet holes not far from his place. Now, I'm starting to become really concerned. The cop informed me that the car was used in a spree of crimes from Friday night until Saturday night ending with the car found in its current condition and is now evidence and being examined for clues as to what may have happened.

Obviously, that wasn't something I was expecting to hear when I went to the police station. Now given the situation he agreed to put out a missing person's report. I was up all night from then on calling his phone that was now just going to voicemail. I decided to go to his apartment and stay there in case he showed up and to get a couple of hours of sleep. Luckily, I recently set up a few of his bills to be paid online with his bank account. I decided to get some sleep and set my alarm for 6:00 am.

When I woke up I logged in to his bank account with his debit card and to my dismay I saw a charge in New Orleans East off of Downman Road which is a hit or miss part of town. My heart immediately sank in my chest as there is no way he should be anywhere near that area of town. Given the fact that his car was used in a spree of crimes and his card was used in the early morning hours in a shady part of town I could only assume the worst. His phone was dead and there was no sign of him. My mind was racing thinking the ones who stole his car may have seen him back with his new rental and took him and the car. What other explanation could there be…

I really didn't know what to do at this point other than pray. A few hours later I logged on again and saw a charge at a gas station in Hammond, LA which is north and west of the city. I got the phone number and called the station but didn't get anywhere with that. A few hours later there was a charge at a fast food restaurant in Denham Springs, LA with was even further west near Baton Rouge, LA and all that time I was called his cell phone that was going straight to voicemail which we all know the older generation tends not to have that set up. I was doing all of this while working… The next time I logged in there was a charge in Slidell, LA which was almost back to New Orleans. Geez!!!

Believe it or not, I was starting to become a little more optimistic that he may be lost rather than dead in the trunk of this rental car. The next day this went on between Slidell and Denham Springs but that evening I was able to track a purchase he made in Independence, LA and the lady at the store said "I do remember him… He came in asking for sweet water and I really didn't know what he wanted but we figured it out and it was Gatorade… Sorry sir I don't know where he was going but he was definitely appeared confused…"

At that point I felt a little better but not great. I contacted the car rental company to see if they could intervene but they informed me that that model does not have a LoJack device on it. Damn… Well, I won't drag this out to long but by the grace of God I was able to track him down to a Mc Donald's parking lot near New Orleans East. He was sitting in his car and when I found him the rental car was a mess with food wrappers, empty bottles, ashes from cigarettes, and he looked at me with such relief I began to tear up… "Dad, where have you been? You ok?... Damn you had a lot of people worried about you…" I could see the frustration in his face, and he couldn't even respond. It was as if he was in shock. I called a Nurse Practitioner friend of mine to see if she could check him out or I was going to bring him to the ER for an evaluation. I really didn't want to put him through that at this point. Anyways, I was able to get him checked out and remarkably he was ok but obviously shook up a bit. He must have had a guardian angel looking out for him. Lost for about 3 days and obviously must have been pulling over and slept in his car. I can't even imagine what he was going through…

It was at that point that I knew I had to start exploring where I could put him. Ultimately, after some trials and tribulations he ended up at the very place he drilled in my head as a kid… A nursing home and he did great! Don't get me wrong, the 1st month or so was a challenge from what I was told be he did well considering. He was about the only one that could walk on his unit, and I think they were a little scared of him lol. He was the Kingpin of the 5th floor! Anyways, he lived a pretty good life for sure. He was able to play with many of the greats like James Brown, B.B King and was on Harry Connick's first album. He was a certainly a character for sure…

As I was about to wrap this up there was one more crazy event that happened that I must mention. In the early morning hours of May 24th 10 inmates from the Orleans Justice Center escaped and the public was not notified until about 7 hours later. What a disaster! Hard to believe… As great as this city can be, it can be as bad as this. When I went back in August of 2023 to document the changes from 20 years ago, I'm not surprised. The inmates were being called residents, which was ridiculous to hear. Here are some clips from this unbelievable event…

https://www.wwltv.com/mobile/article/news/crime/new-orleans-jail-escape/i-should-have-been-the-first-on-the-list-victim-says-he-wasnt-warned-after-escape/289-e448d935-2942-4d71-8662-6cf5f78c83df

https://www.wwltv.com/mobile/article/news/crime/new-orleans-jail-escape/expert-earlier-inmate-transfer-might-have-prevented-jailbreak/289-bb4c8ec5-a6d0-4c9c-a640-8a34c4c6488c

https://www.wwltv.com/mobile/article/news/crime/new-orleans-jail-escape/orleans-jail-escape-arrests-aid-fugitives/289-2c796cab-d4ac-487a-8025-59c39181b20f

It's pretty wild to see all of this unfolding in real time. As of May 21st 2025 there were still 5 inmates on the loose… I guess this will be continued…

Day 7: Five fugitives still missing as new footage, arrests and oversight orders deepen jail escape fallout New surveillance video shows escapees walking downtown hours after jailbreak; governor signs order; defense attorney claims jail worker is innocent

https://www.wwltv.com/mobile/article/news/crime/new-orleans-jail-escape/orleans-jail-escape-day-7-inmate-video-governor-order-jail-worker-inmate-help-civilian-arrests/289-aa387106-3689-4b65-9dab-b96f8deb60dd

WWL+ Special | New Orleans Jailbreak: The first 7 days Our detailed, day-by-day timeline reveals how the escape unfolded and why victims, witnesses, and even prosecutors have now gone into hiding.

https://www.wwltv.com/mobile/article/syndication/ott/wwl-ott/new-orleans-jailbreak-the-first-7-days-wwl-plus/289-ec20a93d-155e-48e7-86fa-564361597ed6Â

Political firestorm grows after Orleans Parish inmate escape Sheriff and DA's office tussle in court over investigation https://www.wwltv.com/mobile/article/news/crime/new-orleans-jail-escape/political-firestorm-grows-after-orleans-parish-inmate-escape/289-9ed65d75-7096-4c24-8b60-733513c52739

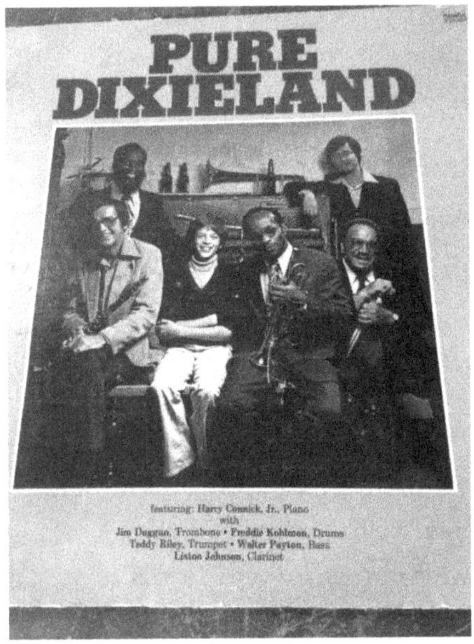

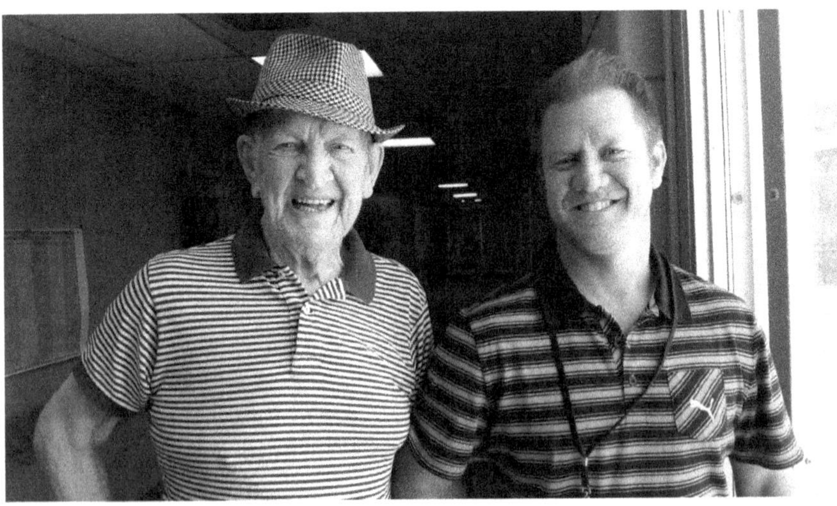

www.ingramcontent.com/pod-product-compliance
Lightning Source LLC
LaVergne TN
LVHW052224200926
848481LV00001B/207
* 9 7 9 8 8 9 9 5 0 1 5 7 9 *